seven 7 steps

TO LONG-TERM CARE PLANNING

Jennifer Crowley

BSN, RN, CLCP, MSCC, CADDCT, CDP

Printed and bound in the United States of America
First printing • ISBN 978-0-9991508-3-2
Copyright © 2017

TO ORDER ADDITIONAL COPIES OF:

seven 7 steps

TO LONG-TERM CARE PLANNING

Jennifer Crowley
BSN, RN, CLCP, MSCC, CADDCT, CDP

VISIT: WWW.SEVENSTEPPLANNING.COM

PayPal

MasterCard VISA AMERICAN EXPRESS DISCOVER NETWORK

Contact Jennifer Crowley: jennifer@sevenstepplanning.com

SC

SCOTT COMPANY PUBLISHING
P.O. Box 9707 • Kalispell, MT 59904
Toll Free: 1-800-628-0212
Fax: 1-406-756-0098

Table of Contents

U-D-E-C-I-D-E

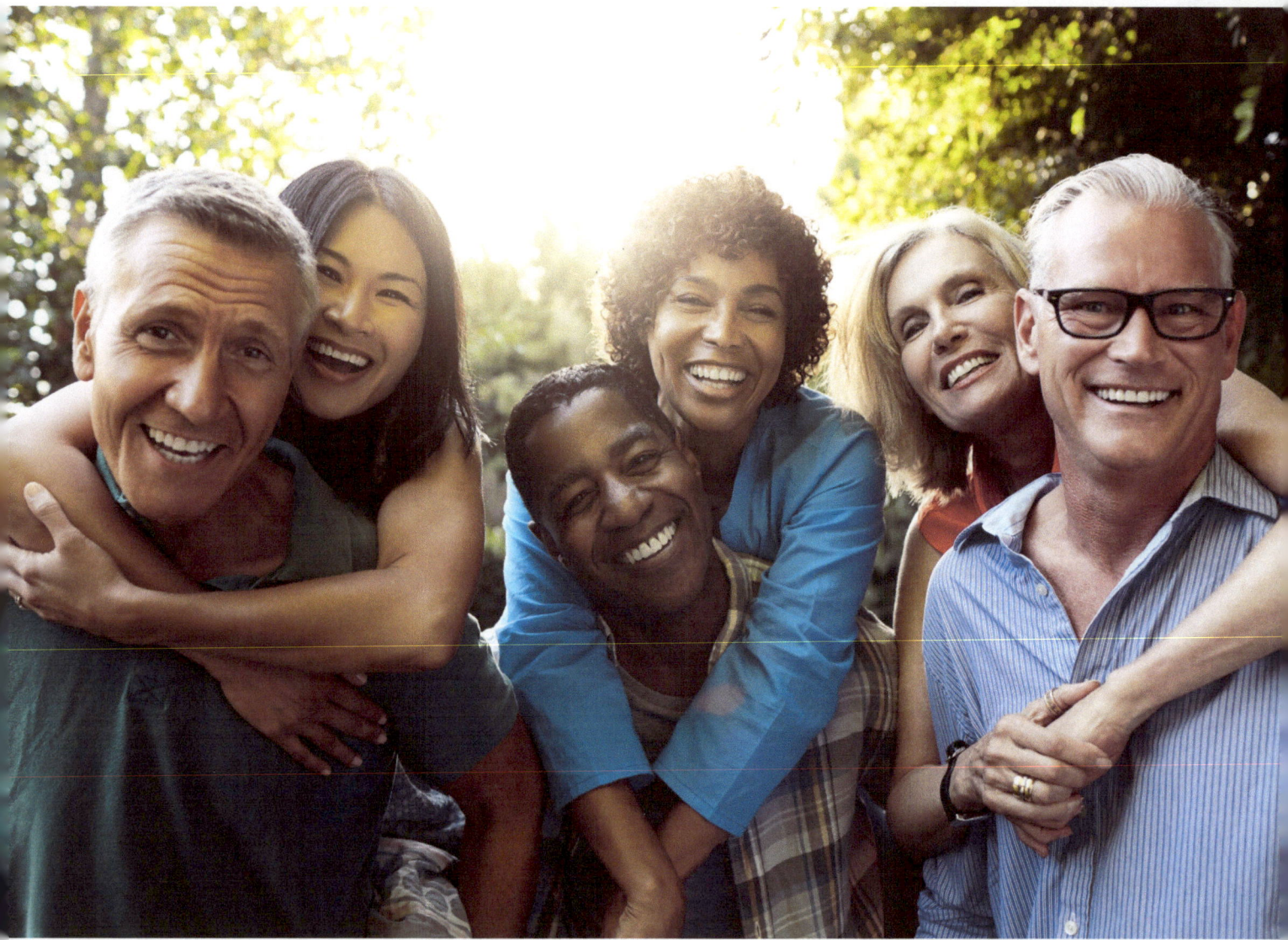

INTRODUCTION

The aging demographics are helping shape how care is delivered and define how communities are prepared. Every day, 10,000 people turn age 65.

People are living longer, often with multiple chronic health conditions that lead to difficulty with day to day life. The number of centenarians, those living to or beyond 100 years of age, has grown steadily and is expected to keep rising. Its is estimated more than half the population of the United States suffers from a chronic health condition.

Living a longer life allows family and friends to learn from their elders, gain valuable insight, and have more opportunities for spending time together. Living longer also increases the chances of requiring assistance in certain areas of life, relying on others to assist with long term care needs. Long term care includes a range of services and supports you may need to meet your health or personal needs. Services may include personal care assistance for tasks of daily living, such as bathing, cooking, transportation, household maintenance, and more. Long term costs rise suddenly with a change in health, such as with an unexpected illness, or with exacerbation of a chronic health condition. Sometimes long-term care needs rise over time, as the condition progresses and normal aging related changes are aggravated by the condition. The aging human body encounters many changes in function through the normal degenerative process that is occurring. There is a general decline in the physical function of the body, including sensory changes with hearing and vision, and decrease in strength and balance, increasing the risk of falls and accidents. A chronic condition may aggravate these normal degenerative changes, making it necessary for lifestyle changes and relying on others for assistance.

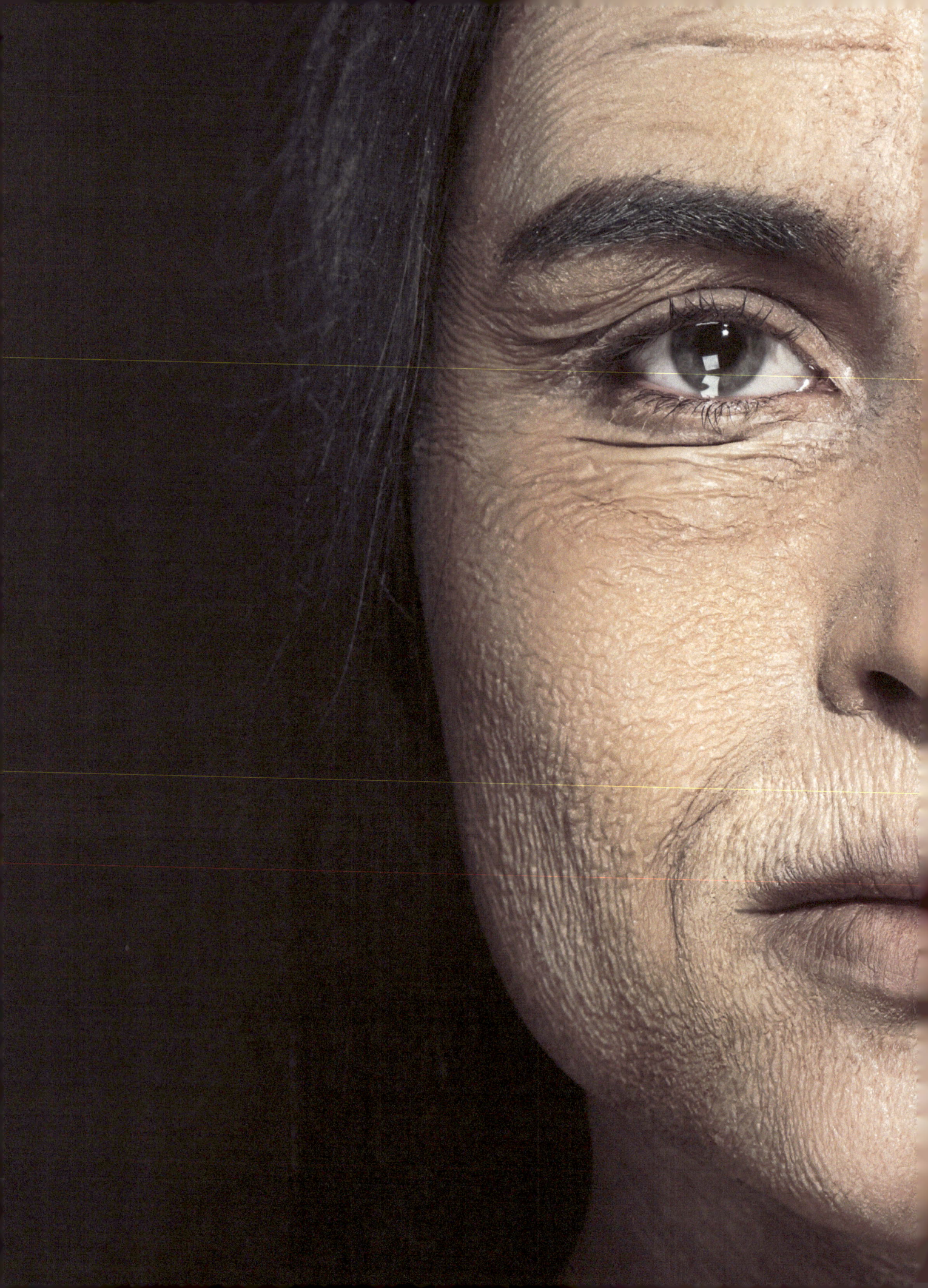

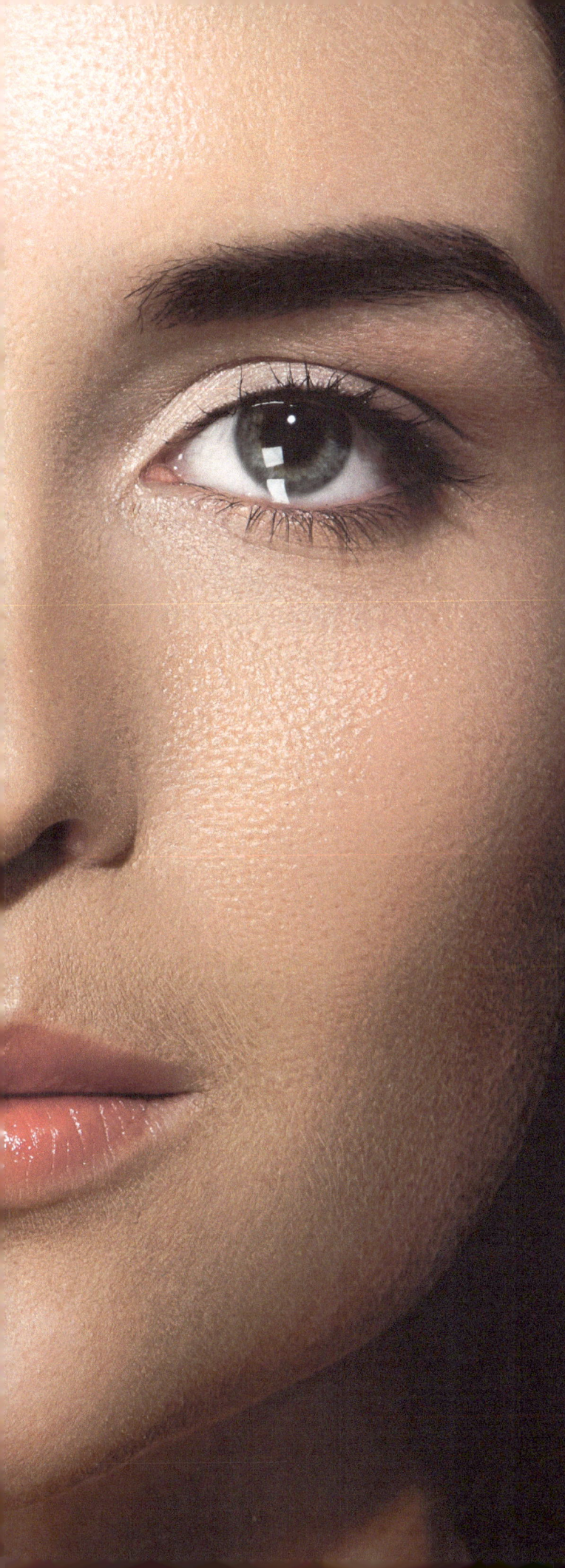

seven**7**steps

TO LONG-TERM CARE PLANNING

Jennifer Crowley

BSN, RN, CLCP, MSCC, CADDCT, CDP

seven*7*steps

A geriatric workforce shortage is taking shape in most communities, causing delays in services and rapid turnovers, resulting in caregivers who may be ill-prepared. There is increased demand for families and friends to take on roles of caregiving, often a role they have little or no experience with. Caregiving is recognized as one of the most difficult jobs, with burn-out and stress reported by most caregivers. Caregiving can be rewarding but have negative consequences, impacting the health and livelihood of the caregiver. Caregivers report numerous challenges to one's physical, emotional, and financial well-being. Caregiver stress is well recognized in many policy decisions with insurers, including Medicare, which has a benefit option for allowing caregivers to receive respite, or a short break from their caregiving role.

Aging demographics and associated issues threaten communities and governments on a global and local level. The challenges are many. Communities and governments are promoting aging friendly agendas with many towns creating programs to enhance or add services. Relying on funding through government sources and private donations often fall short for communities to be able to provide services in a cost-efficient manner. The reality is that planning for long-term care is highly personal and the responsibility of everyone. It is important for individuals and family to engage in meaningful discussions early and have a plan. Failure to plan for potential care needs, an unexpected illness, or medical emergency often leads to crisis decision-making, greater dependency on paid professionals, and potentially limited options.

The greatest challenge in preparing a long-term care plan is knowing where to start. This guide will help you get started and create your road map for aging. It is not too late to get started. Sometimes things happen before we have a chance to act. For most of the over 5 million Americans living with

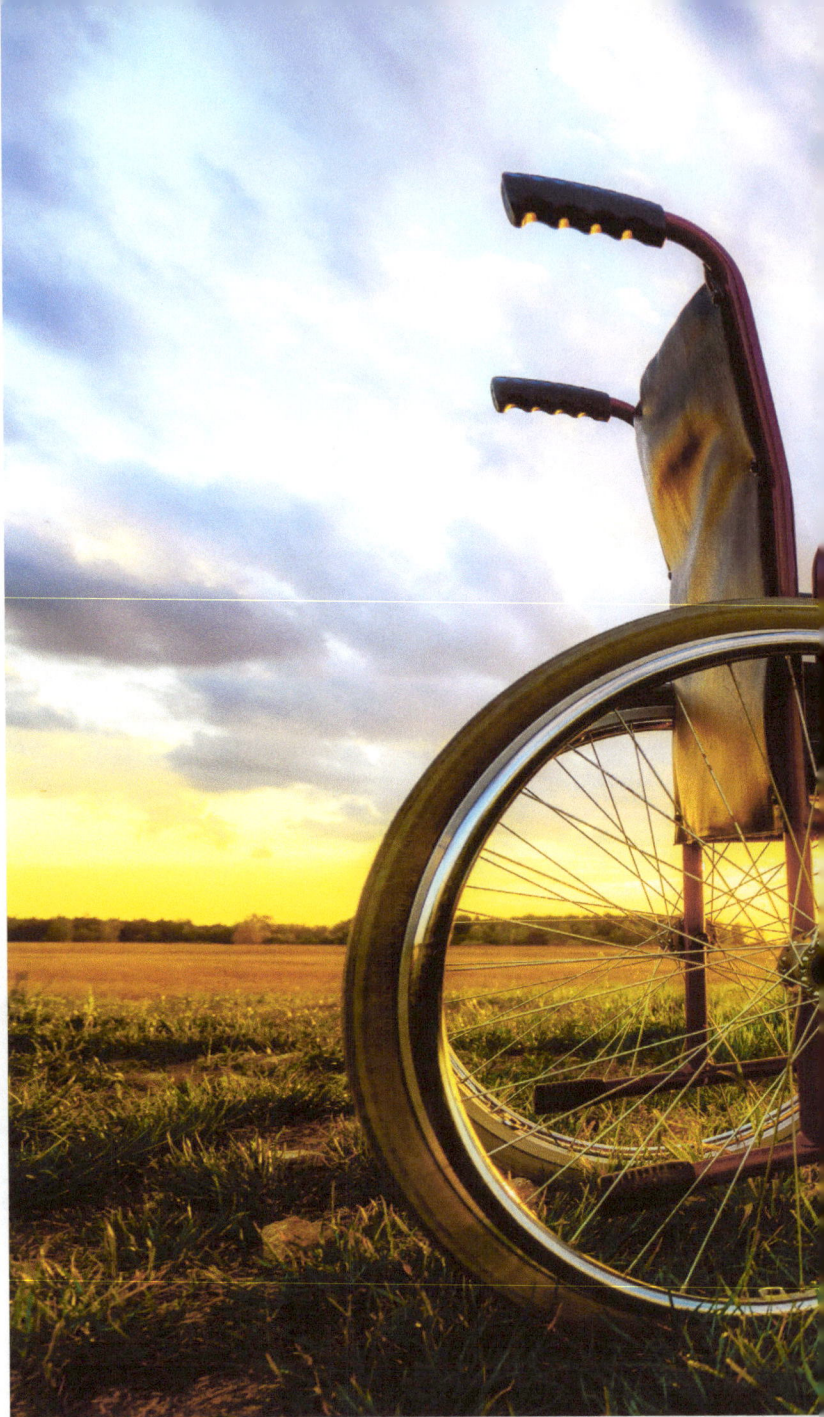

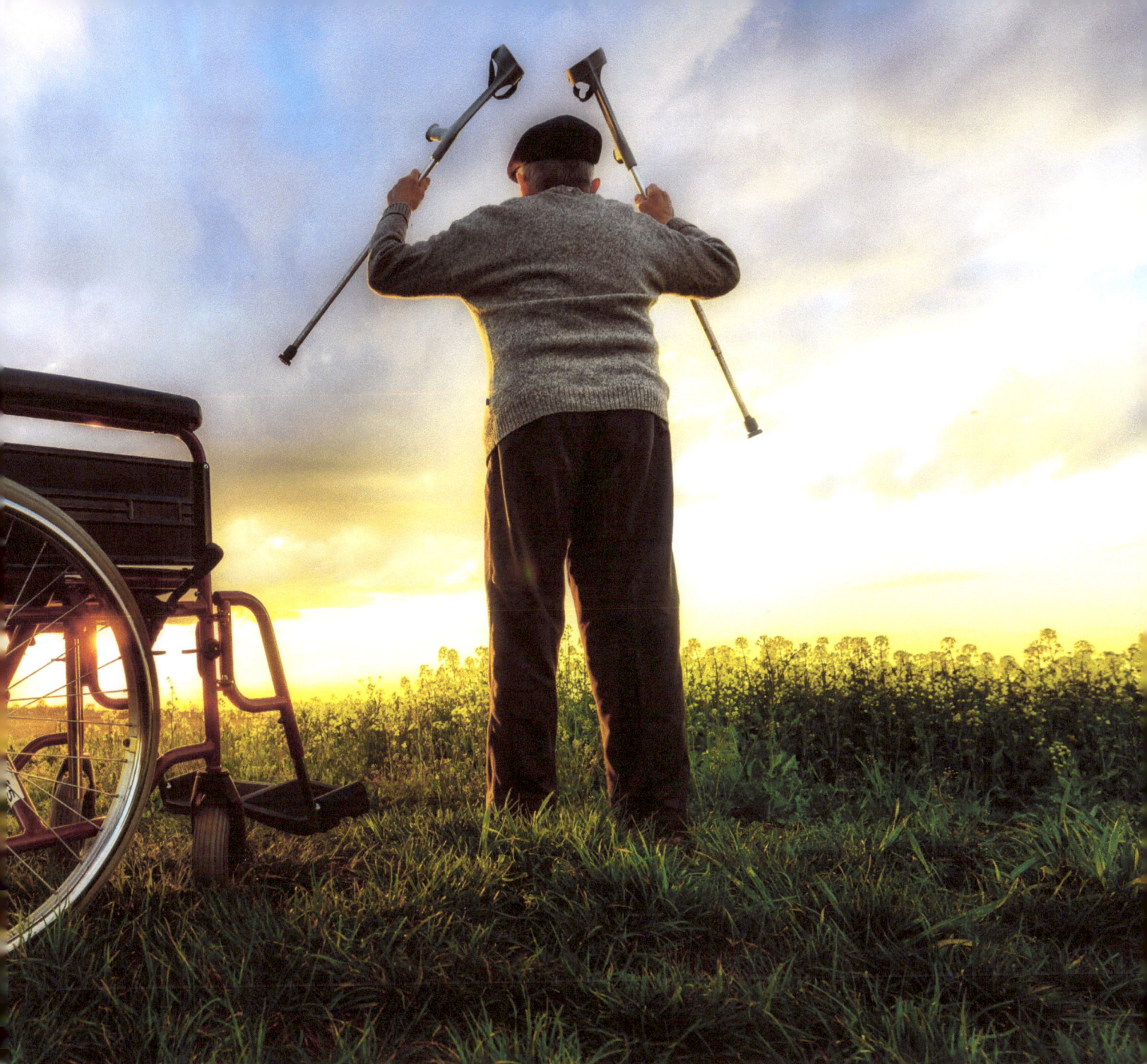

Alzheimer's disease or Related Dementia, a diagnosis came late, after memory loss had set in and difficulty with decision-making became apparent. With cognitive impairment, the individual needs to act swiftly to be a part of the decision-making process, ensure their wishes are protected, and their affairs are in order. A failure to plan early can result in a tremendous financial and emotional burden, and the deterioration of the person-centered approach. There should always be a quest for making your wishes known, needs met, and having the most desirable, appropriate road map for aging.

This guide will move you through a simple 7 Step process for working through difficult conversations and making informed decisions. You will gain valuable insight while developing your road map for aging, regardless of your situation. You will avoid crisis decision-making by utilizing this 7 Step process. It is comprehensive but simple and to the point. The goal is for your peace of mind and sense of control, so you can focus on the joyful parts of life.

It is easy to understand what you want out of life. The more difficult task may be understanding truly what it is you need. As we age, things may get more complicated. Maybe you suffered an injury during your youth or young adulthood which is now aggravating normal aging related changes. Perhaps you have acquired or been diagnosed with a medical condition which is anticipated to be chronic, or long term, and progressive in nature. This first step is typically the most difficult; that is, truly understanding what the needs are. I often hear in family member's voices the distress they feel from not knowing where to begin or where their situation is headed. If this is you, you're in the right place.

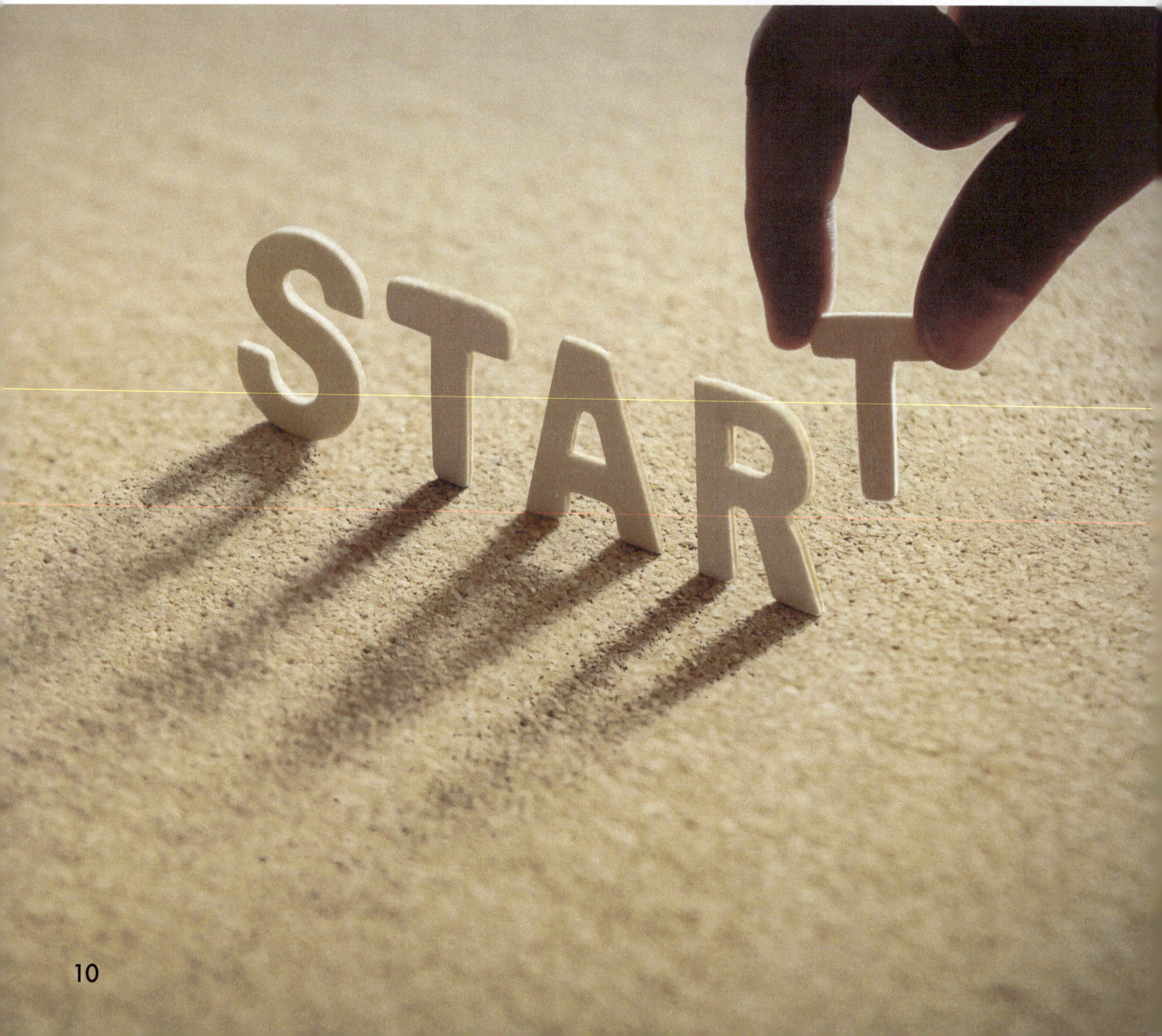

This first step typically takes the longest. Don't be discouraged. It takes time and mental energy to focus on your situation. Remember, you do not need to complete all 7 Steps in one day or one week. You took the first step and that is often the hardest step to take.

Maybe it's more straightforward for you. That's good. For many, starting here is like uncovering rocks and looking for clues. The clues you might be looking for are sometimes buried deep and not written down. It's okay. Take this first step and I'll try to make it easy for you.

Medication Review

A good place to start involves understanding the routine medications and the reason each medication is taken. A review of all medications a person is taking is referred to as medication reconciliation, considered standard of care for improving safety by helping reduce adverse drug events and medication errors. Once a review of the regular medications is complete, the health conditions or diagnoses often become more apparent. It is disappointing to learn someone is taking a medication for which they have no understanding of their reason for taking it. But this is common. Use the information below to help answer some questions which may reveal the actual diagnosis or reason for taking the medication, as well as focus on special items to consider when reviewing a medication regimen. A helpful form is provided for your use on page13.

There may be more questions after reviewing this information. This exercise will also help you identify questions to discuss with your physician.

Questions may include:

- Who is the prescribing physician?
- How long has this medication been taken?
- What are the potential side effects?
- Are there any special items to consider? Special items to consider include the risk of taking the medication due to interactions with other medications, dietary considerations, or if the medication needs to be taken in a special manner.

It is important to review the safety of medication administration and the way the medication regimen is adhered to. Contact your pharmacy and ask to speak with a pharmacist to assist with this process, if necessary. Most pharmacists will help you review each medication and what it is used for as well as things to look out for.

Important Questions:

- Are medications organized and in a safe place with visible instructions on each bottle?
- Is a list of the medications always available and kept up to date?
- If more than one physician or health care provider is involved, do they all have the same list?

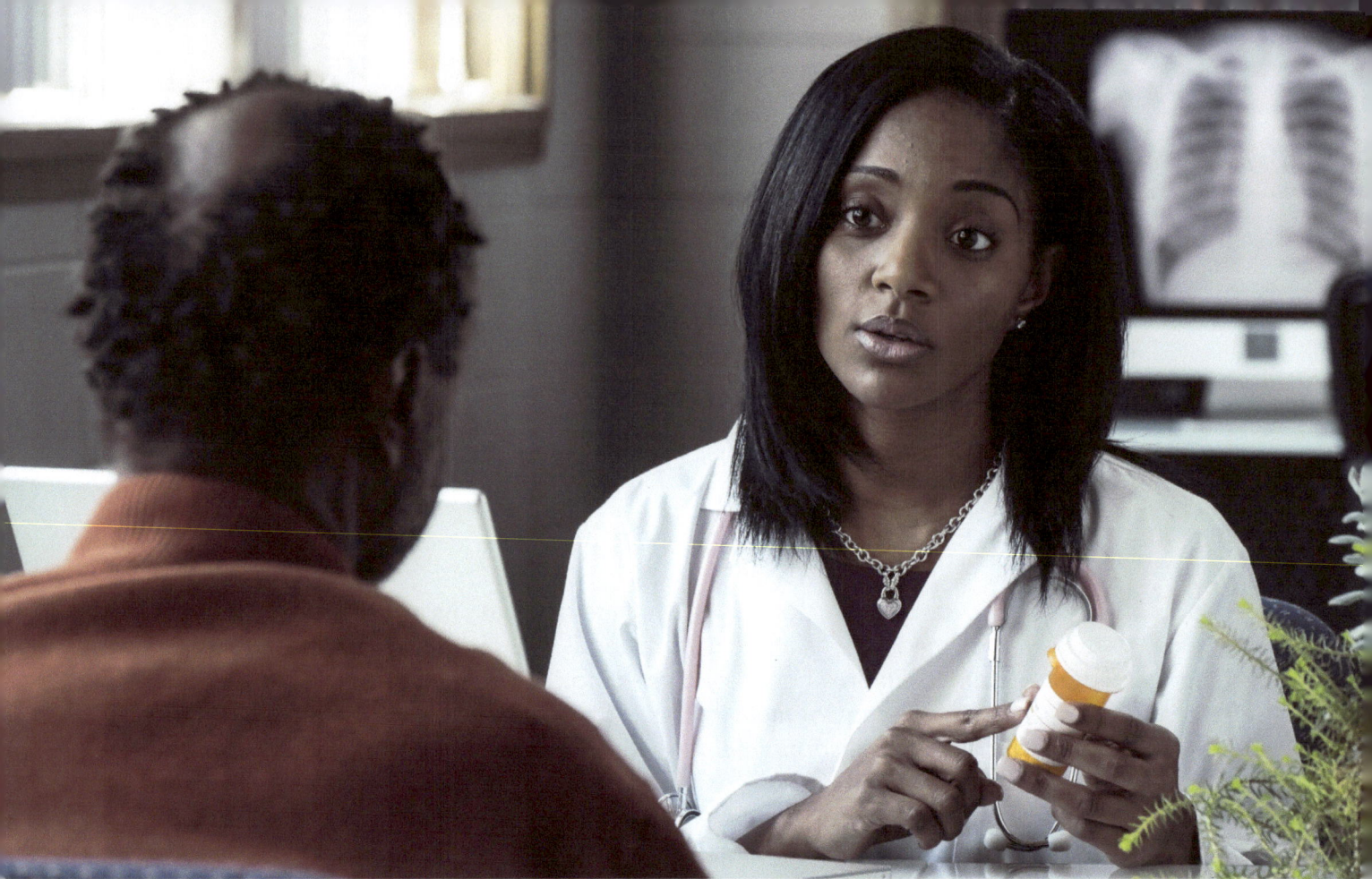

Sometimes medications are organized in a pill box, allowing for daily dosing without opening each bottle every day or multiple times per day. Other methods include having your pharmacy prepare a blister pack. A blister pack organizes the daily medications in a "blister pocket" which is opened daily. The medications are removed from each corresponding day's pocket, providing a simple mechanism for tracking adherence. This method is not available at every pharmacy.

Other methods for medication administration include automated dispensers, programmed by the user to deliver medication at a certain time per day. With these devices, alarms and notices are sent to registered individuals to notify if a medication is missed. It is important to have a reliable method for medication administration since this is an area with a high incidence of errors, potentially causing unnecessary hospitalizations and complications.

Review the method the medications are administered.

Answer these questions:

• Are medications taken as prescribed without reminders?
• Have you been known to forget to take your medication?
• If you need reminders, how does this occur?
• Is there a daily alarm or other form of electronic reminder?
• Is there a loved one or caregiver who reminds you to take your medications?
• If a pill box or pill organizer is used, who sets that up and makes sure it is refilled?
• Are there certain behaviors or memory issues which make it difficult for someone to understand their daily medication routine?

Use this form to document the routine medications. Be sure to include over-the-counter medications, those which do not require a prescription. Vitamins, supplements, pain relievers, or other medications used infrequently but to treat a minor ailment should be included.

Medication	Dosage or Amount	How Often or Frequency	Time of Day	Reason for Taking the Medication	Special Considerations or Side Effects to Look for

Health Status

Now that you have taken a close look at medications, you should have a clearer understanding of what conditions are being treated. Expand on what you learned by moving into a review of all conditions. A list of the most common conditions is provided to assist you.

Utilize the list of conditions provided to identify important questions about your health status or that of a loved one. If you have ever sought treatment for any condition(s) or have one of the conditions which is managed by a medical provider, it is important to have this documented. If you are not certain then be sure to call your medical provider's office and request your medical records. Most individuals don't know they can do this but it can very enlightening to review your own health record. You may learn something which is very important.

Most providers will release records to you, if you sign a release for information. This can be mailed or faxed to you if a provider is no longer caring for you, has your pertinent health records, and you are living at a distance from them. While this may seem cumbersome, it is typical for health care agencies and provider offices to refuse direct handout of medical records due to their "ownership" of the records. Although the records are about you and your health or that of your loved one, the information within the record is protected health information through federal law, the Health Insurance Portability and Accountability Act (HIPAA). Many health care agencies have on-line web portals available for sharing your electronic health records with you, with the customary security and user agreements.

It is estimated more than half the population of the United States suffers from a chronic health condition. Older adults take at least 2 medications routinely to help manage a chronic condition or prevent one from occurring. As we age, the likelihood of this increases as the degenerative process is aggravated by health conditions or injuries.

Here is a list of common conditions which may be considered chronic in nature, lasting greater than 6 months, and progressive, meaning it may become more problematic as time goes on. Use this as a guide to help you complete your list of medical conditions.

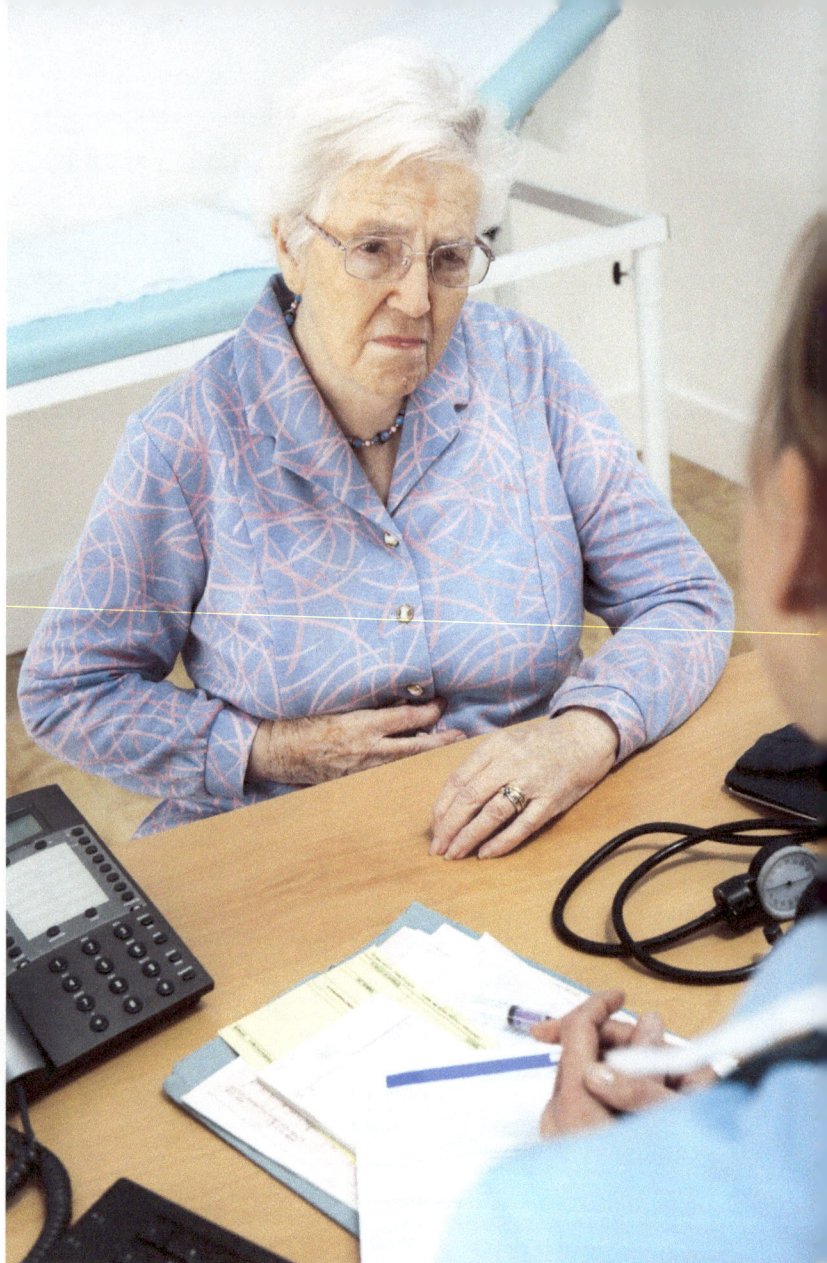

List of common health conditions:

o   High Blood Pressure

o   Obesity

o   Heart Attack or Coronary Artery Disease

o   Congestive Heart Failure (CHF)

o   Arthritis

o   Stroke

o   Cancer

o   Back or spine condition

o   Chronic Pain

o   Peripheral Vascular Disease

o   Depression

o   Diabetes

o   Other mental illness or disorder (schizophrenia, bipolar, manic-depressive)

o   Anxiety

o   Chronic Kidney Disease

o   Parkinson's Disease

o   Hypothyroidism, or under-active thyroid

o   Multiple Sclerosis

o   Dementia

o   Mild Cognitive Impairment

o   Amputation of extremity or digits

o   Organ Transplant

o   Neurological Condition

o   Auto-Immune Disease

Medical Condition or Diagnosis	When was it Diagnosed? Not sure? Provide an estimate.	Symptoms related to medical condition	Treatment Plan For example, diet, medications, daily weights, write what you know

Now that you have completed the medication and condition lists, focus on the day to day activities and review if assistance is needed in any manner to fulfill those daily tasks. Day to day tasks may seem mundane and something each of us fail to put much thought into or take for granted. The health care industry refers to the day to day tasks someone must accomplish to care for their body and environment as Activities of Daily Living (ADLs) and Instrumental Activities of Daily Living (IADLs). With certain conditions, the performance of ADLs and IADLs become more difficult, requiring assistance on a routine basis. This step involves taking a closer look at the current situation to help understand what the current needs are. Later, we will move through the process for review of potential or anticipated future needs. This may seem difficult but start by learning a bit more then utilizing the form provided.

Activities of Daily Living include:

- Bathing
- Toileting
- Dressing
- Mobility-moving your body from one place to the next. Examples: walking, wheel chair dependent, use of walker
- Transferring-moving your body from one position to the next. Examples: independent, hands-on assistance needed to get up from chair, requires lift for getting in and out of bed or in and out of a vehicle
- Eating-the task of getting food from the plate to your mouth or ability to drink from a cup.

Instrumental Activities of Daily Living include:

- Shopping
- Housekeeping
- Home Maintenance
- Meal preparation
- Transportation
- Setting or making appointments
- Using the telephone
- Use of household appliances
- Finances
- Social participation
- Exercise

Types of Assistance can include:

- Cueing or Instruction to initiate the task
- Supervision for safety, someone at arm's length during the task
- Hands on Assistance to complete the task
- Total Dependency
- Combination of one or more above

Assistance with Activities of Daily Living is typically carried out by the immediate family and is referred to as personal care assistance and include tasks that are custodial in nature. Tasks may require assistance by outside help depending on the situation. Certified home health agencies provide short term help in the home following an injury or accident. This skilled level of home health services

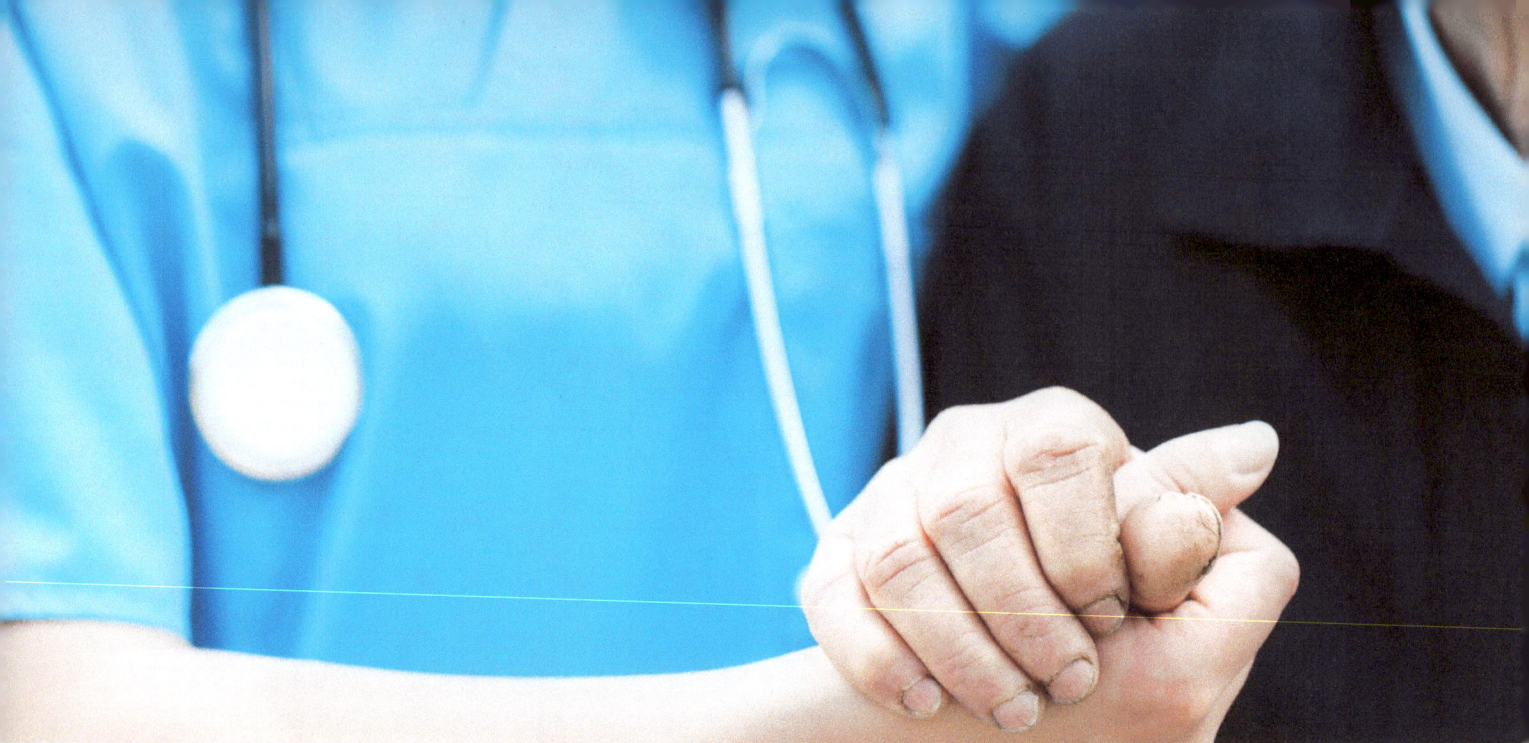

requires a doctor's order and is covered by most insurers. Skilled Home health is usually provided by licensed professionals such as Physical Therapists, Social Workers and Registered Nurses. It is typically short in duration and dependent on the individual to meet goals and demonstrate progress.

Long term care in the home which is custodial in nature, and does not require licensed professionals, is considered non-medical personal care assistance. Home health in this capacity is typically provided by non-licensed professional caregivers, such as Personal Care Attendants, Certified Nursing Assistants, or Home Health Aides. It is important to understand what the current home health plan is and whether it is sufficient to meet the needs of the individual. Most individuals and families elect to have personal care assistance to alleviate the demand for their time and help keep their loved one safe while they are away. Others may live alone and need to hire help to remain in their own home.

Long term care in the home and personal care assistance may be provided by:

- Family caregivers, the Informal unpaid caregiver
    - o Spouse or Partner
    - o Daughter
    - o Son
    - o Sibling
    - o Others
- Paid caregivers or other health care professionals through an agency
- Paid private caregivers, hired independently and privately
- Volunteers through community partners
- Friends or neighbors
- Pastoral or faith based supports
- Certified home health agencies

Determine if help is required currently and how much time is provided for each task. For example, if bathing assistance is required, how often is help provided and how long does it take to complete the task of bathing?

Use the table below to help provide a snapshot of current needs.

Activity/Task	Help needed to complete? If YES, complete additional columns	What type of help is required	How often is help needed	How much time is provided to complete the task	Who provides the help
Bathing					
Toileting					
Dressing					
Mobility					
Transferring					
Eating					
Shopping					
Housekeeping					
Meal Prep					
Transportation					
Setting or Making Appointments					
Using the telephone					
Using of Household Appliances					
Finances					
Social Participation					
Exercise					

Bringing it all together

Having a clear understanding of your current situation is helpful for being able to move through the next steps. Even if your situation involves perfect health with no reliance on others to assist with your personal needs, it is still meaningful to move thru the 7 Step process. It is important to review your wishes and consider important topics to design your personal road map for aging, helping to prevent crisis decision-making and avoid adverse outcomes.

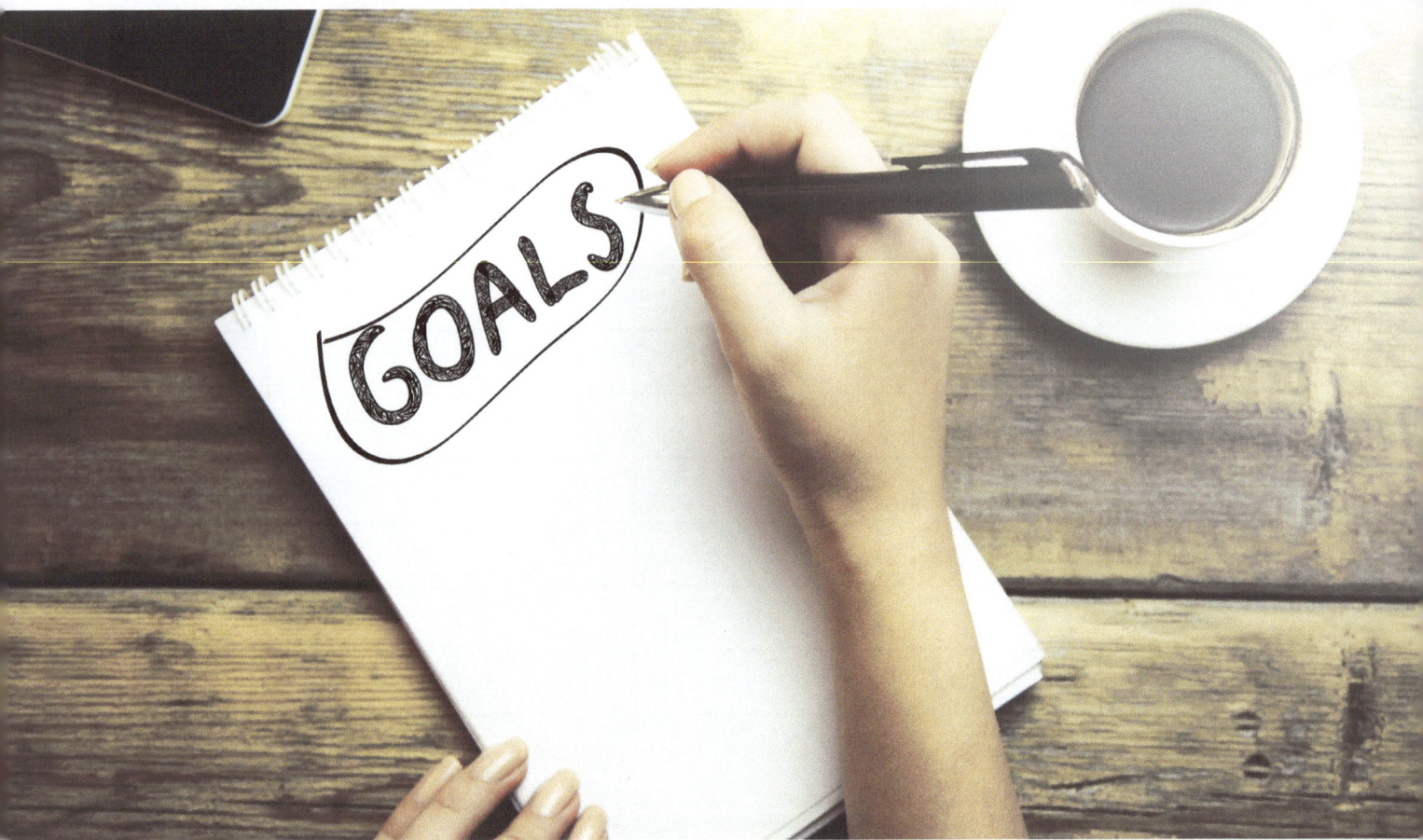

A goal can be defined as the outcome or achievement toward which effort is directed. Setting goals focuses your attention on the desired outcome and helps direct your actions. Goal setting is important for improving self-management and improves healthcare providers' ability to provide person-centered care. Most human behavior is goal-oriented. Meaningful activities are designed to achieve some type of outcome.

In this step, we will also focus our attention on a topic which is very important, legal documents. Often, these are not completed, leading to potentially costly outcomes. Legal documents, including Advance Directives are recommended to any adult, and strongly encouraged for anyone living with a chronic illness, disability or cognitive impairment. It is important to complete legal documents early and review them often especially as situations change. This is a logical item to include in this section. Start your list of goals in this step, or actions you wish to take to reach your desired outcome and design your road map for aging. If you have not completed your legal documents or you have not reviewed them in the last six months, this should be your first item to include on your goals list.

It is important to note that Step 2 is fluid in nature, meaning you can come back to this step as needed, to add to your list of goals at any time and review them or make notes. A form is provided to help you track your goals on page 27.

To help you learn more and develop a consistent method which can be applied in all areas of your life, we will review the S-M-A-R-T method. The S-M-A-R-T method for setting goals can even be expanded to include two additional steps, making it S-M-A-R-T-E-R. This is a well-known method used by professionals across many disciplines, including professional care managers, social workers and business leaders. Many successful leaders make a list of their goals regularly and return to their list to determine if they have achieved what they set out to do and what course of action may be necessary, if any. You don't need to be perfect. We all have experienced setting out to do something with good intentions and things getting in the way, making it difficult to complete our task at hand. The best leaders fail regularly but have a system for re-setting and re-strategizing. Let's learn about the method which can improve your chances for success and provide direction as you design your road map for aging.

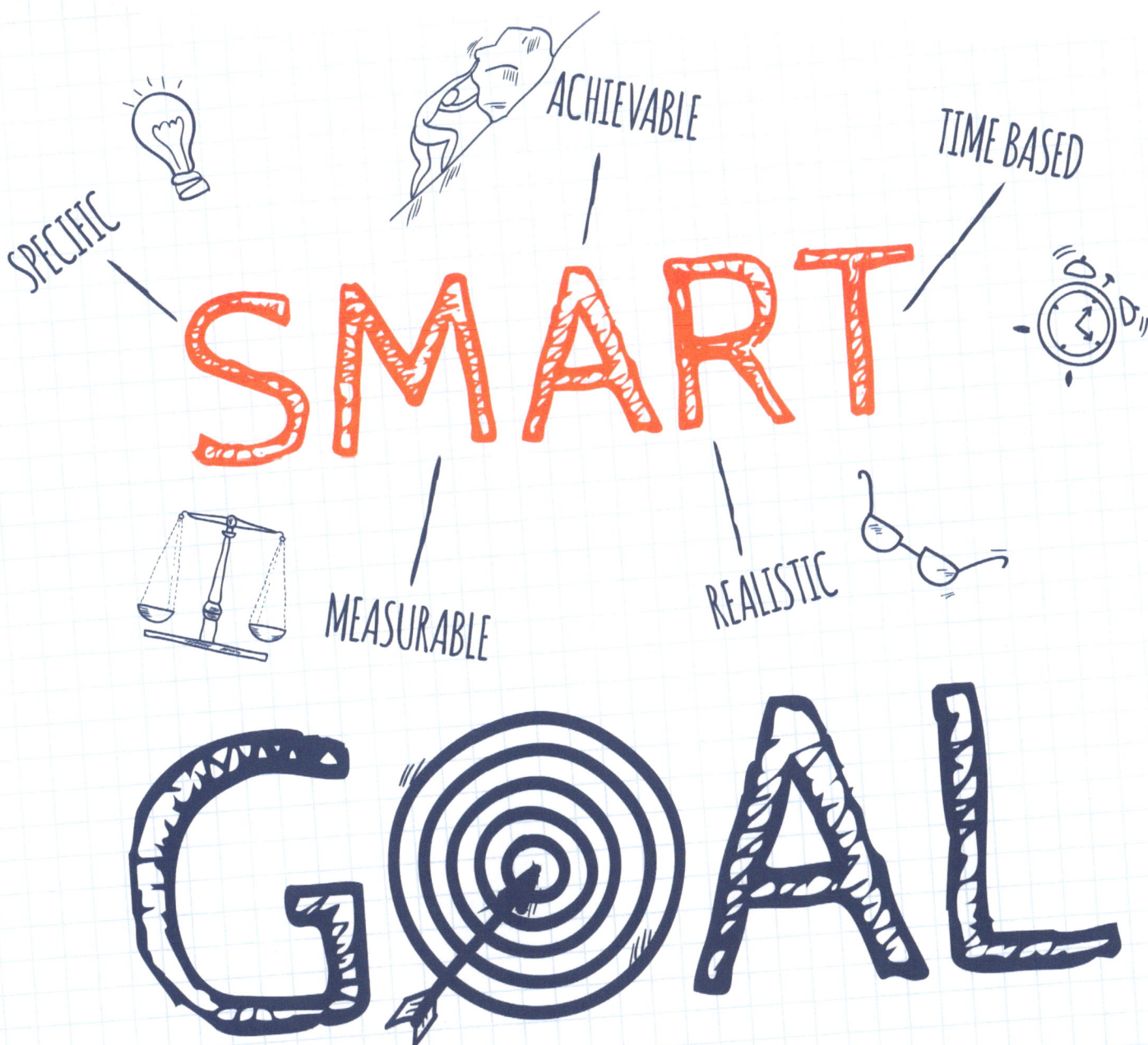

SPECIFIC

ACHIEVABLE

TIME BASED

SMART

MEASURABLE

REALISTIC

GOAL

The steps for use of the S-M-A-R-T-E-R method for setting goals:

1. Specific
Create a simple goal and be very specific.
It should be clearly identifiable.

2. Measurable
Create a way to check if you are making progress you anticipated.

3. Achievable
A task or action which is possible, capable of happening or within your grasp

4. Realistic
Consider if it is too lofty or too difficult for you to accomplish. Ensure success by not creating too lofty of goals or ones that are nearly impossible.

5. Time-based
Give yourself an end date or time for completion of the goal.

6. Evaluate
Review your goals and change or modify the goals if your situation has changed. Evaluate your progress and re-set your timeframe for completion, if necessary.

7. Re-evaluate
Conditions and situations may change, creating a need to re-evaluate your needs and reset your goals. Through accomplishment of goals comes a sense of control, empowerment, and preparedness.

Next, we will review legal documents. Legal documents are highly recommended to have completed when designing a road map for aging. After reviewing this information, move to the form for listing your goals and include the appropriate legal document which needs completed or reviewed, one at a time. Keep it simple and don't forget to add a timeframe for completion.

Legal Documents

No long-term care plan is complete without addressing the legal mechanisms for protection of your wishes and direction for those involved in your care or management of your personal affairs. The legal documents best suited for an individual will depend on the situation, family and state laws. Consultation with an attorney is always encouraged and highly suggested, depending on the complexity of your situation. Most states have access to legal documents recognized as valid and reliable, typically found on their web site.

In general terms, here is some information to help guide you through what to expect and documents you may wish to consider:

- **Decision-making:**
  Who will make decisions for you or act on your behalf to manage your personal affairs if you are not able for some reason?
  This is typically identified as a "proxy decision-maker," or someone who can ensure your

wishes are protected and your needs met if you are incapacitated for some reason. Ideally, this is done early, prior to any decline in health or onset of cognitive impairment. If done early, the completion of legal documents pertaining to decision-making authority does not require a doctor and some documents can be done without an attorney. Most documents must be signed in front of a notary. Once a person is no longer able to participate in decision-making due to memory loss or difficulty processing complex decisions, a costlier approach may be necessary. This may include the need for obtaining legal guardianship and conservatorship, which typically is done through the court system and requires multiple legal professionals to be involved as well as participation by one or more health care professionals. This will vary depending on state laws. Words of caution: Make sure to put extra thought into who you will give authority to for handling your personal affairs or helping make healthcare decisions in the event you cannot do this yourself. Ideally, the individual is a family member in good standing, not in financial or other crisis, or with failing health themselves. Most documents can be revoked in case something changes but be sure to review who is best fit to act on your behalf if it becomes necessary.

Legal Documents to consider:

Power of Attorney for Health care

Power of Attorney for Financial

Guardianship and/or Conservator

What happens if you don't designate a proxy decision maker or give authority to someone to act on your behalf if you cannot make decisions?

Most states defer decisions to the next of kin starting with a spouse, adult child, or sibling. This will vary depending on the situation and the family structure. It is important to make your wishes known and designate a person to act on your behalf.

• **End-of-Life or Advance Directives:**
If you were to require life-saving measures, are your wishes well known and documented? Does your family and provider understand what you want in the event your heart was to stop or you were to stop breathing?

These decisions are very personal and involve a health care provider. Typically, an attorney is not required for completion of Advance Directives. However, if you work with an attorney often be sure to let them know your wishes and ensure they have on file a copy of all your important documents.

Legal Documents to consider:

Living Will

Physician Order for Life-Sustaining Treatment (POLST) form

Do Not Resuscitate

Five Wishes

- **Last Testament & Will**

Designed for after your death, instructions include what to do with your estate or personal possessions and how to manage your affairs. This is typically done by an attorney and will not be elaborated on here. However, if an attorney prepares a last testament and will for you, they often complete Power of Attorney and Advance Directive documents at the same time. This will vary depending on the professional and state laws. In most cases, there is an executor of the estate designated, the person who will take care of the matters related to your estate once you are deceased. This is typically a family member but can be a close friend or sometimes an attorney. Make sure to pull out your Will and review it and make changes as necessary.

Laws and customs pertaining to healthcare and financial decisions will vary depending on each state. Individual state laws impact how an estate is managed by someone else in the event the individual is no longer able to manage their own affairs. If your situation is complex or you have difficulty with finding suitable resources to understand your specific needs, consultation with a professional such as an attorney is recommended.

Developing goals provides focus toward achieving your desired objective or anticipated outcome. Through accomplishment of goals comes a sense of control, empowerment, and preparedness.

GOAL

Now that you have learned about the S-M-A-R-T-E-R method for setting goals, let's do an example of how to apply it to your own situation. We will apply this method to completing a legal document which gives authority to an individual to make decisions-the Power of Attorney for Health Care, as this is the most common deficiency in my long-term care planning experience.

This is often the first goal, set right away when designing a road map for aging.

Let's apply the method we learned, using this example:

1. Specific
"I will complete a Power of Attorney for Health Care document in 30 days."
This is specific and to the point. This includes a deadline.

2. Measurable
What are the items you must achieve along the way to complete this goal?
These are considered targets or interim milestones along the way.
For example: Obtain the document from appropriate source (state web site, aging services, attorney); choosing your proxy decision maker; speaking with family; or making an appointment to have the document notarized, if appropriate.

3. Achievable
These documents are available and straightforward. You got this!

4. Realistic
This document requires some careful thought but is straightforward and can easily be completed. It is not lofty or unattainable.
It is realistic to assume you can complete this document. You can do it!

5. Time-based
"I will complete a Power of Attorney for Health Care document in 30 days, <set date here>"

6. Evaluate
Look at what you accomplished!
This is a good time to review the document, decide if anything has changed, including the status of the person you just gave authority to in the event you are unable to manage your health or finances.

7. Re-Evaluate
Do this periodically, such as every 6 months to determine if your situation has changed.
Decide if any changes need to be made. If not, rest easy. You did it!

NOTES:

Use this form to help you set your own goals and track your progress through completion:

What do you want to accomplish? (make sure this is realistic and achievable for you) GOAL:	How will you measure your progress? Milestone towards progress:	When will you complete this goal?	Date of completion:	Re-Evaluate every 6 months. Changes? No changes?

step 3 EVALUATE WHAT YOU WANT

It is important to take the time now to evaluate what you want and what your vision is for your aging life. The steps in this book are grounded with a methodology designed for a person-centered approach. This step places significant attention on the individual. Focus is placed on the individual's likes, dislikes, attributes, wishes, and personal situation.

This step is very personal, thought provoking, and often emotional. Sometimes we have failed to think of ourselves as an older person, too confused about what that means and difficult to imagine what our life will be like. Certain situations arise making it difficult to achieve what you want.

Sometimes, what you want no longer matches what you need, creating a need to cope with the adjustment and make changes where necessary.

When this process is applied early, strategies may be developed for your situation, helping you to accomplish what you really want. The longer you wait to decide, the more difficult it may become to identify the means for achieving what you want. If you are trying to decide what someone else wants, because they can no longer tell you what they want due to Dementia or some other condition, the burden is real and it can be very hard. As you move through this process you will begin to understand how to identify with the wants and desires for yourself or your loved one(s).

If you are helping design a road map for someone with cognitive impairment who can no longer state their wishes or participate in difficult decision-making, try taking the time for reflection on the past. Reflect on moments when that someone mentioned their wishes, dreams, or desires for their aging self, prior to their cognitive decline. Perhaps you had conversations about others who were going through changes in health or experiencing a situation necessitating a need to plan quickly. Did they ever mention what they would want if they were in a similar situation? Sometimes wishes are clear but most times they are not, due to the personal nature of the topic. This reinforces the need to have legal documents complete and up to date, early.

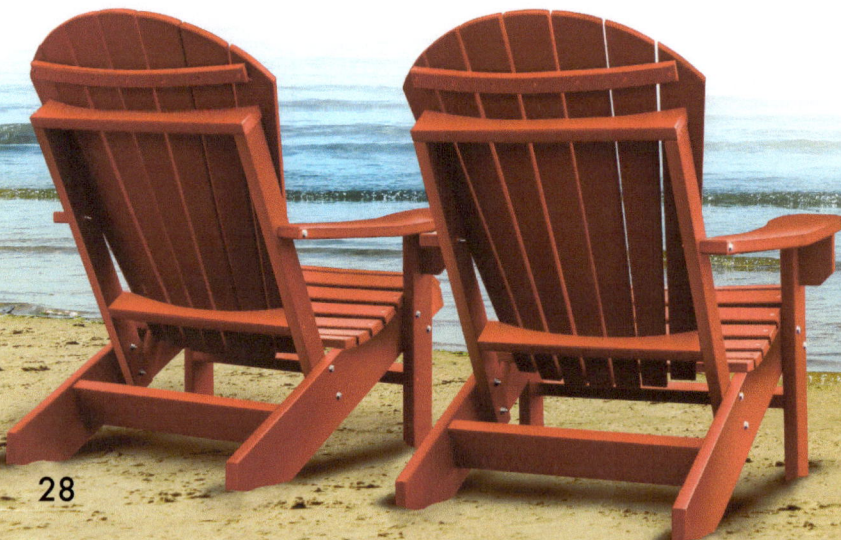

Here are some questions to help you move through this step:

- How did you see yourself as an older person?
- Do you have plans for where you will live?
- What is your aging in place plan?
- Are there family members who can take care of you if you need it?
- Are you opposed to living in "senior housing", assisted living, or residing in a nursing home?
- Do you plan to transition to an older adult community at a certain age?
- Is it important for you to stay active and get regular exercise?
- Do you enjoy nature or being outside a lot?
- How important is it for you to be close to family?
- Have you always been concerned about being a burden to your family as you grow older and may need more help?
- Have you always expected to travel as an older adult, enjoying culture and the arts along the way?
- Do you wish to age in a cold or warm weather environment?
- Did you always want to live as long as possible, no matter what?

NOTES:

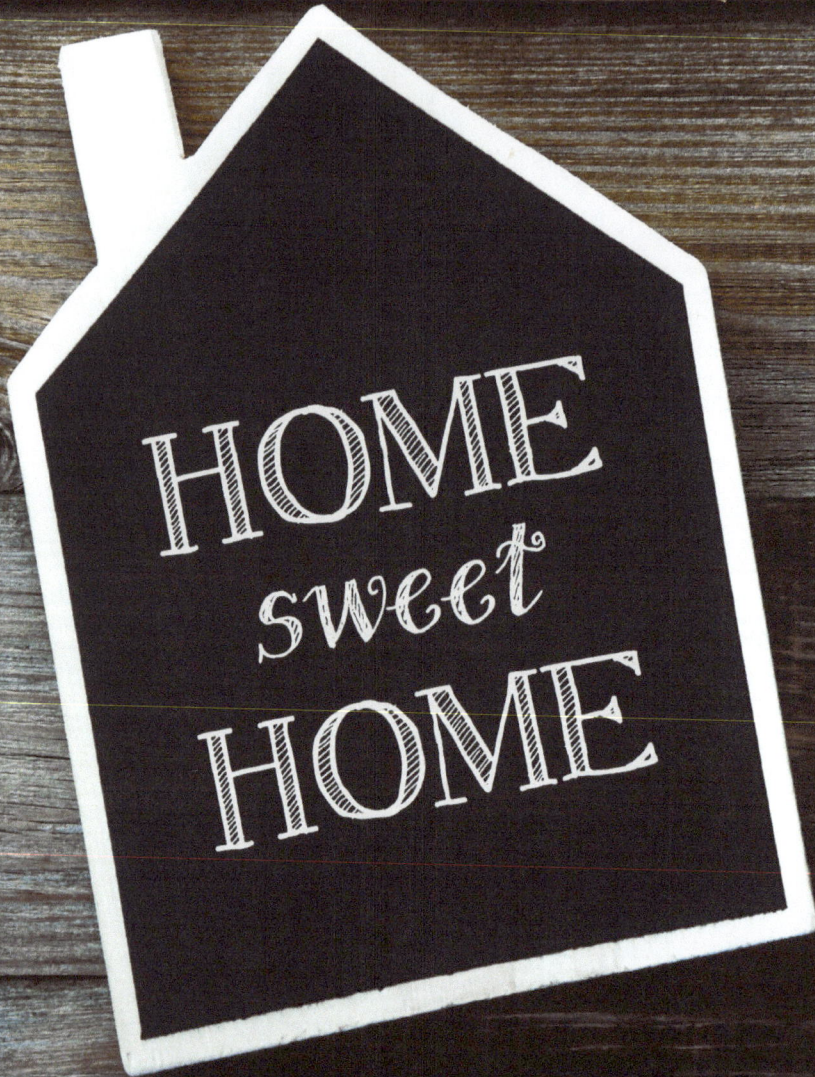

The most important component of the aging in place plan is the suitability of a home to meet the needs of an aging adult. In this step, we will focus on the Aging in Place plan. While most communities recognize the need to design streets and buildings according to the Americans with Disabilities Act (ADA) guidelines, most homes in America require modifications and renovation to improve independence and safety with aging, failing to prepare communities to face our nation's changing demographics. A disability home renovation to accommodate for a change in health status or aggravation of normal aging related changes can be very costly. Some homes cannot be modified without structural changes and significant burden of time and cost and dust.

Universal accessibility refers to a structure, such as a home, being accessible to all, regardless if they are a resident or a visitor. Residents and visitors to that home, regardless of ability, can enter and exit the home and carry out activities of daily living using the primary living spaces. Primary living spaces are areas utilized to carry out the necessary functions of life, such as bathing/toileting, dressing, sleeping, meal prep/eating, and should include an area for socialization or activities. An Aging in Place plan in the home should include a careful review of the primary living spaces and their suitability for carrying out activities of daily living while maintaining safety and promoting independence.

When reviewing the primary living quarters of a residence, one must keep in mind the floor plan and the ease to which someone can move from room to room and whether mobility devices can be used effectively and safely, if it becomes necessary.

Questions to ask when reviewing your Aging in Place plan include:

- Are there steps into the home?
- Are doorway thresholds difficult to navigate?
- Are the door ways wide enough?
- Are handles easily manipulated?
- How many steps are required to enter or navigate the home?
- Where are the primary living spaces located?

I often encounter homes with the primary living spaces on the second level of a home, making it challenging for the older adult to maneuver steps, especially while carrying objects. Residential homes come in all shapes and sizes and are frequently added onto or modified for the needs of a growing family. However, additions and changes to the home are not always done with aging in mind and placing careful thought into the ability to remain in the same home through end of life.

With aging, there is a decrease in balance and strength. Any chronic health condition, especially with the use of multiple medications to manage the various conditions, can contribute to aggravation of normal aging related changes. Statistically, older adults take two medications routinely. Medications, as discussed in Step 1, have side effects and interactions which may contribute to increased falls or decreased ability to entirely self-manage a condition. This reminds us the importance of understanding all the medications someone is taking in the home and the potential side effects, so that extra vigilance can occur and safety measures within the home are completed in a timely fashion.

Often, families are faced with the decision whether to do a construction project or plan for a transition to a facility for their loved one. Careful consideration with retirement planning may improve your ability to remain in your own home.

Additional questions include:

- What is the bathroom like?
- Does the bathing area have an easy step in or roll in shower?
- If there is not a suitable bathroom, can one be added or renovated easily?
- Are grab bars or some type of support rail able to be installed in key areas?
- Is there a handheld showerhead and available shower bench?
- Are services available close to the home if it becomes necessary?
- Are there supports in the immediate area if help is needed or to keep a helpful, watchful eye if necessary?

It is important to remember safety equipment is useful for not only the person needing help but for those who are providing direct caregiving to that individual. Any tool a caregiver can use to help another adult is useful and appropriate and may include such items as a gait belt, raised toilet seat, grab bars and hand-held showerhead. Simple measures can be taken to improve independence with functional tasks as well as promote safety.

A solid aging in place plan includes goals to:

- Promote Independence
- Improve Safety
- Help the individual remain in their own home thru end of life

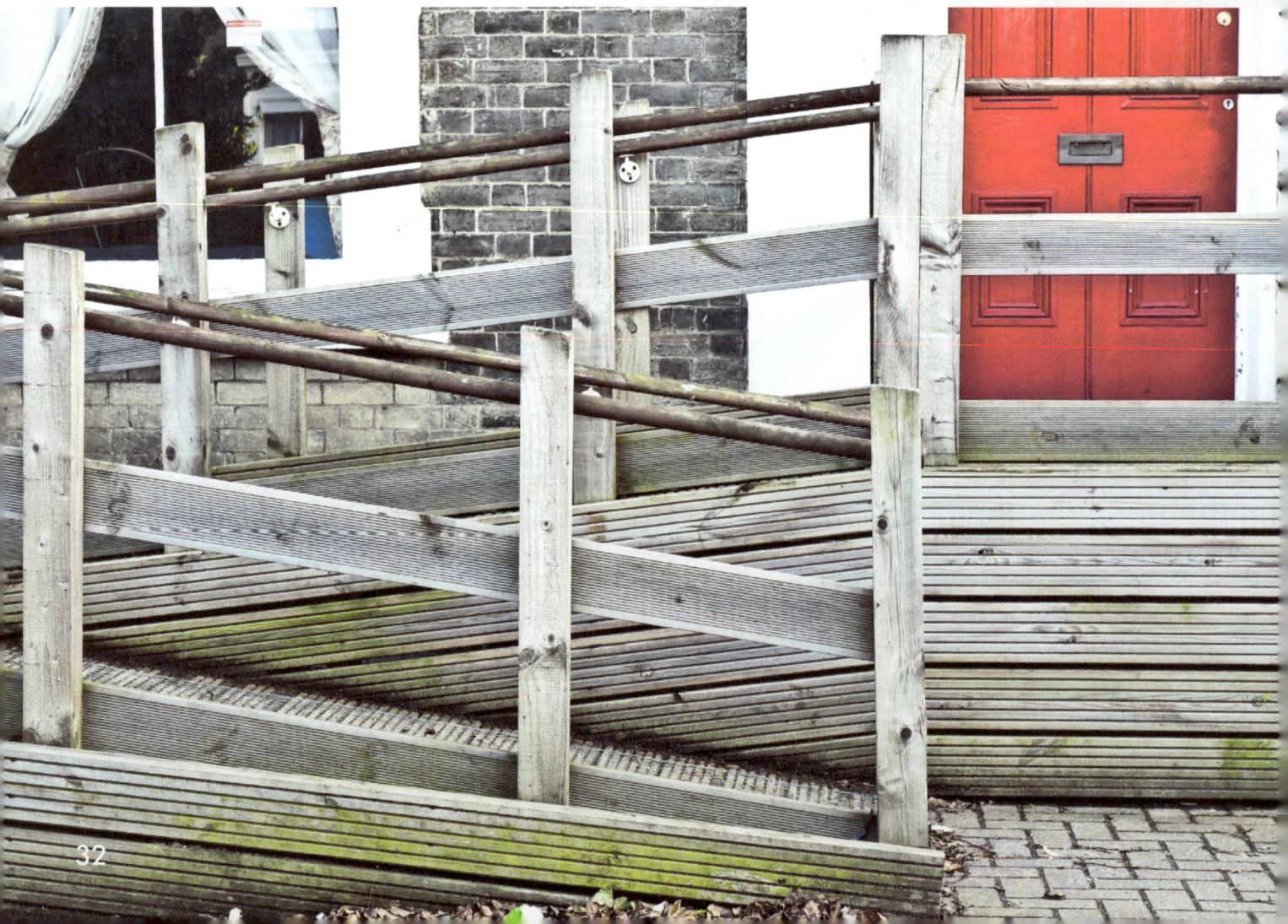

An aging in place plan may include a:

• Plan for transition if home becomes not suitable or less desirable
• Plan for transition if personal wishes include living a simpler life with easy access to services if necessary
• Plan for transition if care needs demand a higher level of care than what is available

Consultation with a professional who specializes in home safety evaluations may be necessary. A home evaluation can be completed, helping to review the primary living spaces and identify areas of concern and make recommendations for changes to improve safety and function.

What if the home is not suitable for Aging in Place through end of life?

The residential home setting may not be suitable for optimal health and wellbeing for the aging adult, necessitating a plan for a transition. This is often the case for someone living with chronic illness, disability or cognitive impairment. There are many reasons for this.

This may be due to:

• 24-hour care being required, creating high demand and complicated scheduling
• Not enough available staff or caregivers to meet the needs of the individual
• The individual can no longer be cared for safely in their own home
• A wheeled device is necessary, creating difficult access
• Entry to the primary living space involves steps which are not easily navigated anymore
• Residence is remote and far from services
• The individual lives alone and relies on paid help
• Safety concerns
• Residence too large to care for any longer

When an individual requires help in the home routinely, they often rely on family members or friends and may need to hire help to provide adequate supports and breaks (respite) to the usual caregivers. There is currently a geriatric workforce shortage taking shape across America. Shortages of caregivers and health care professionals is predicted to increase. This may necessitate a plan for a family to move an elder into their own home or develop an alternate plan. Some families can make the necessary changes to the home because their needs are not complex, more a matter of safety and surveillance. Maybe the changes are small, such as with the addition of equipment such as grab bars and a hand-held showerhead. They may choose to do a costlier renovation or remodel to improve accessibility and function. The typical cost of a disability home renovation can be as high as $15,000. Many families cannot take on the cost of undergoing a construction project, often electing instead to strategize and plan for a transition to a facility or alternate residential setting.

In Step 7, we will discuss exploring services within your community, such as assisted living, memory care, and other options. Completing all the steps is necessary for truly understanding your situation and being able to make the best-informed decision on what is right for you and your family.

step 5   IDENTIFY CAREGIVERS

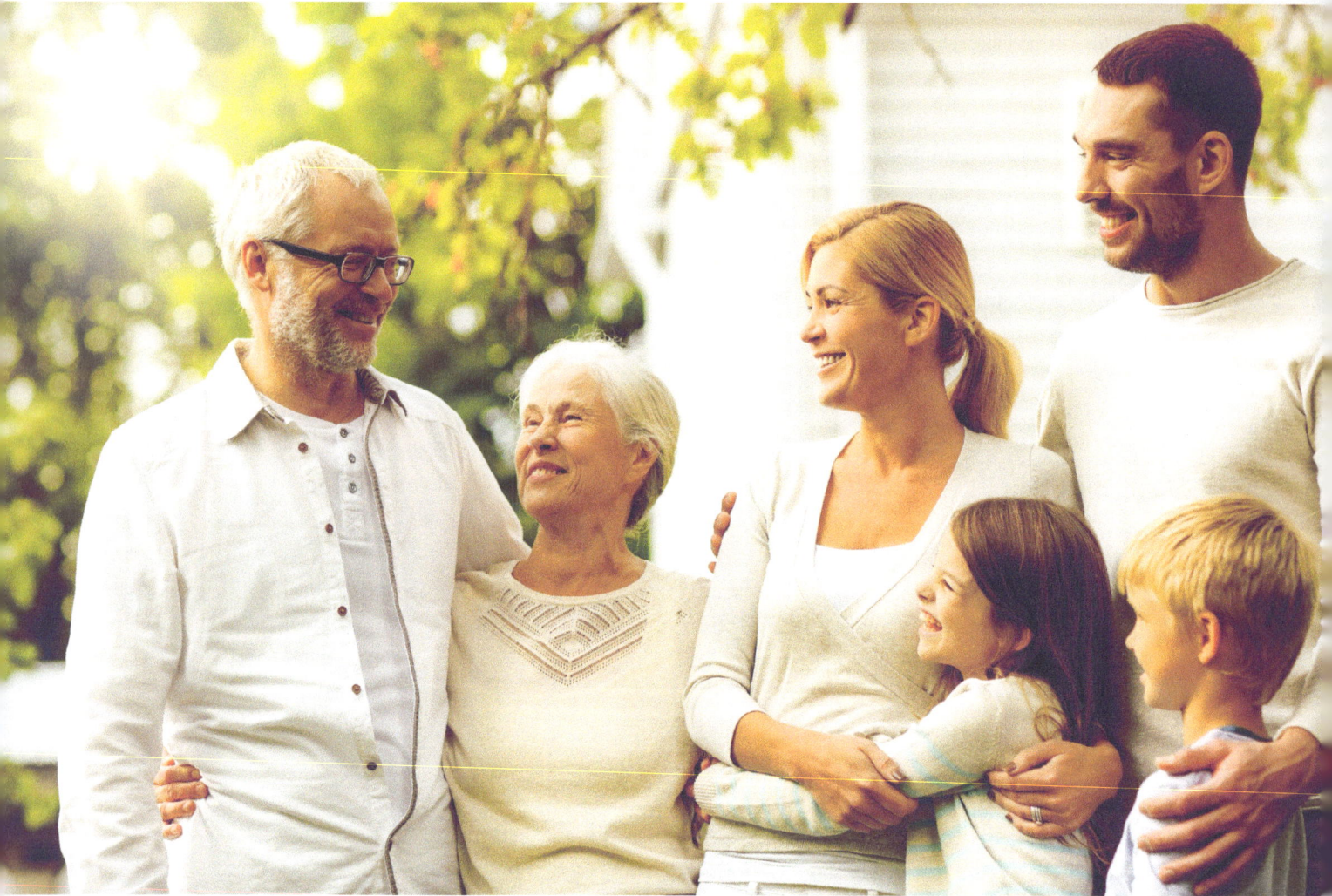

This step focuses on the unpaid support team, the informal or family caregiver.

The first action is to recognize those who are already providing support and assistance. If you currently are receiving help from someone, this should have been addressed in Step 1. Add each person who provides assistance to the list provided with step 1, no matter how small their role or how little time they may spend helping you. These are your informal caregivers, your "village," and part of your home health team. In most circumstances, this is unpaid help provided by family members.

If you are not currently requiring assistance, it should be anticipated at some point you will likely require help with one or more activity of daily living as you age. If you do have help, perhaps your situation is changing or you recognize a need for more help. Not all older adults require help as they age but statistically speaking, if you are living with a chronic health condition that is progressive in nature and requires daily management, it is not a matter of if you will need help but rather when. A diagnosis of cognitive impairment, such as with Alzheimer's Disease or Related Dementia, raises the certainty for the need for 24-hour supervision for safety and assistance in many areas of daily living. It is important to plan for this need and do it early.

Start by making a list of your potential helpers. This list will focus on the unpaid caregivers in your inner circle, the ones who may help you maintain financial security for longer and remain in your home safely and happily through end of life. Let's face it. Home health care is expensive. Most individuals are not prepared to pay upwards of $50,000 per year for personal care assistance. A sustainable, financially sound plan is to include unpaid caregivers on your home health team.

The list should include your most trustworthy relatives, identifying those who have your best interest in mind. Use the form provided on page 5 of this section to help you complete this step. The list should include individuals who may be able to assist you, either occasionally or routinely. They are your team, your support system, the village we know it all takes sometimes. Frequently, the informal or unpaid caregiver is a spouse followed by children and other family members. Sometimes friends or neighbors become an important part of a team to support someone in their own home.

Consider moving outside of your comfort zone. Most humans are not interested in sharing their deepest wishes nor exposing their limitations. Sometimes you just need to consider the day you may need help or face the reality that you really should ask for help.

When reviewing family or friends for a potential caregiving role, make sure to take the time and review what all you know of them. Use the helpful information on the next page to review characteristics of a successful caregiver.

Characteristics of a successful Caregiver:

- Trustworthy
- Good relationship history
- Reliable
- Patient
- Flexible
- Sense of Humor
- Responsible
- Self-directed
- Commitment to a team
- Positive Attitude
- High self-esteem
- Willingness to learn or adapt
- Able to care for others without constant reward
- Financially stable

Red Flags & Warnings!

The informal caregiver to avoid is or has:

- Abusive or abuse history (verbal or physical)
- Short-tempered, angers easily
- Under financial stress or in significant debt
- Dependent on you for financial security
- Excessive use of alcohol or drugs
- Has health problems of their own which are complex
- Has poor relationship history with you, past grievances or arguments
- Attention seeking or needing constant reward or gratitude for small chores
- Has difficulty being motivated
- Difficulty working with others
- Has stolen money or other important items
- Unreliable or unpredictable
- Currently caring for others at the same time (young children, other adults requiring assistance)
- Unwillingness to discuss care with others

It is important to understand not every person can provide caregiving support. It does not mean they are not decent and compassionate human beings. Every individual is unique and for some it is difficult to provide care to others. It really depends on their personality, their upbringing and experi-

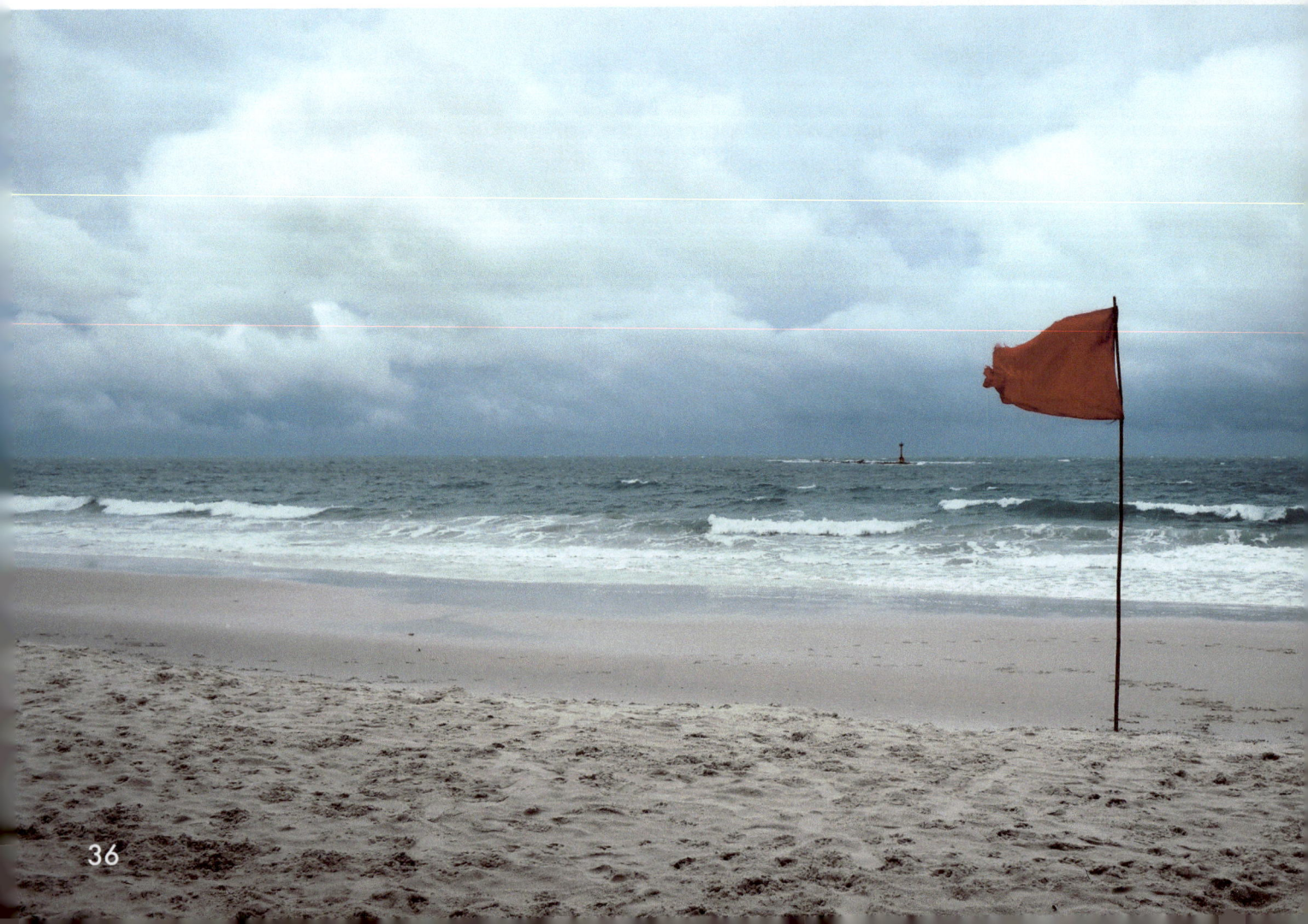

ence. The experience of having been a caregiver to someone certainly helps but it does not always translate to the best outcome. Caregivers, whether paid or not, require some training or at the very least should be completing self-directed learning and be able to take advice from professionals without feeling picked on. Being open to learning about caregiving and learning new strategies or tips can be very helpful. Often, care that is considered substandard, or neglectful, is related to the caregiver having not received adequate training or education.

Neglect may or may not be intentional.

Substandard care that is considered abusive or demonstrating neglect will typically cause negative outcomes for the individual receiving the care. Most often, it is directly related to the caregiver being forced into the caregiving role without being prepared or meeting the characteristics of a successful caregiver.

Substandard care may result in:

- Depression
- Dehydration
- Malnutrition
- Incontinence
- Immobilization
- Pressure sores
- Rough handling
- Poor Hygiene
- Frequent infections
- Withdrawal from activities or socialization
- Isolation
- Medication errors
- Frequent hospitalizations

Consider the power of education and ensuring your caregiving team is sufficiently prepared to handle the job at hand.

COMMUNITY

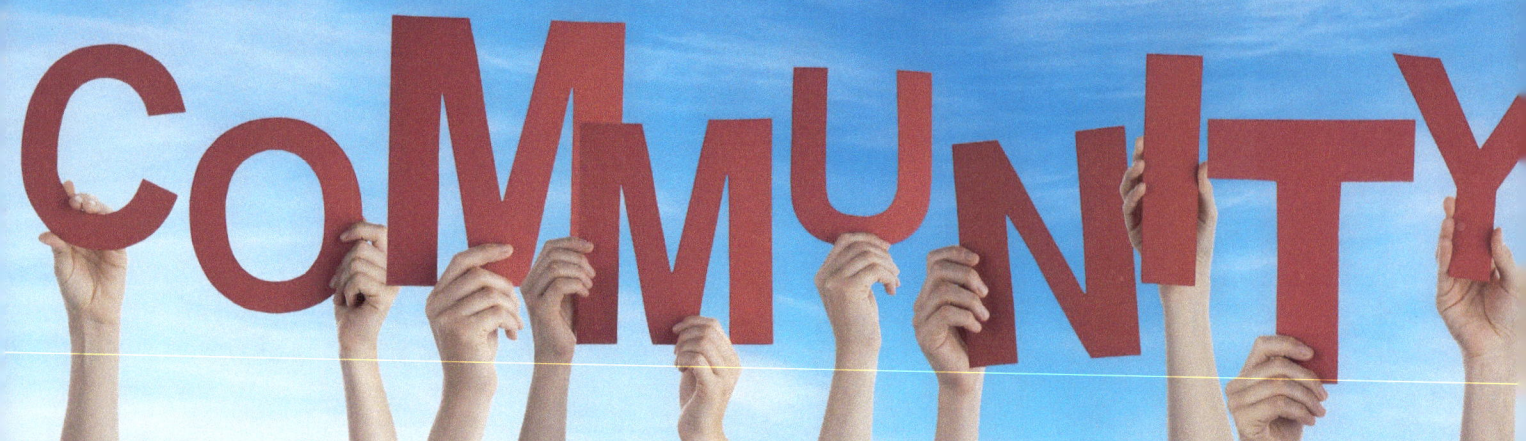

Additional resources for cost-efficient or free help may be available in your community. This will vary depending on your geographic location and available services. Increasingly, services are in high demand but not readily available due to lack of funding or other issues, such as workforce availability. Communities embracing an aging friendly platform look at alternatives to government funded programs and work to develop key partnerships with other organizations to maintain, enhance, or add valuable services.

Other options for creating your informal home health team, beyond family & considering your community resources:

- Faith based organizations with volunteers for transportation, visits, or errands
- Aging services that offer programs for providing respite breaks or other services
- Senior Centers with members who regularly help with various tasks and offer meal assistance
- Meal delivery program to improve nutritional status and offer passive surveillance and monitoring through regular, established visits
- Volunteer organizations

After completing your list of potential caregivers, consider your needs. If your needs are current, a good time to discuss your situation with those on your list is now. Open the door to helping them understand your situation and getting on board to help. It is good to confirm with those who you think can help. Determine if they are still available and interested, or if their situation has changed. Americans live extremely busy lives and although most are caring and want to help, many are caught up in their own careers and families to be able to offer any consistent caregiving. We've all heard the "call me to get together" or "call me if you need any help" statements from friends and family. The truth is we all move through life at an extremely fast pace. The invitation still stands but sometimes you need to provide a mechanism for truly making it happen.

Use of calendar is helpful when discussing your situation with your team. Getting a commitment to a certain day of the week on a regular basis helps you enjoy more days and plan for your needs accordingly, as well as your joyful pursuits. It also allows your caregivers to schedule their time appropriately and hold them accountable. If your informal supports fall through on their ability to meet your needs, then perhaps a review of your situation and where your needs can best be met should take place. If your situation does not include any family or friends who are available to help you as informal, unpaid caregivers, you should anticipate requiring outside help from paid caregivers. In Step 7, we will review how to evaluate and choose paid service providers.

Use this form to help make your list of potential and current informal, unpaid, caregivers

Name	When are they available Day of week/time of day	Special Notes or Instruction

step 6 DETERMINE FINANCIALS

One of the most determining factors in improving your choices and options with respect to your long-term care plan is related to your financial portfolio. Having the financial means to pay for your care means freedom of creating a road map for aging that is aligned with what you want and what you need instead of having to suffice with only what you need.

Do not underestimate the need for early financial planning for long term care

Why worry?

Long term care includes services devoted to assisting someone with their activities of daily living which are typically considered custodial in nature, or those required for the general upkeep and well-being of a human. A common misconception is government will pay for long term care. Unfortunately, most payor sources such Medicare and other insurers consider custodial care to be the responsibility

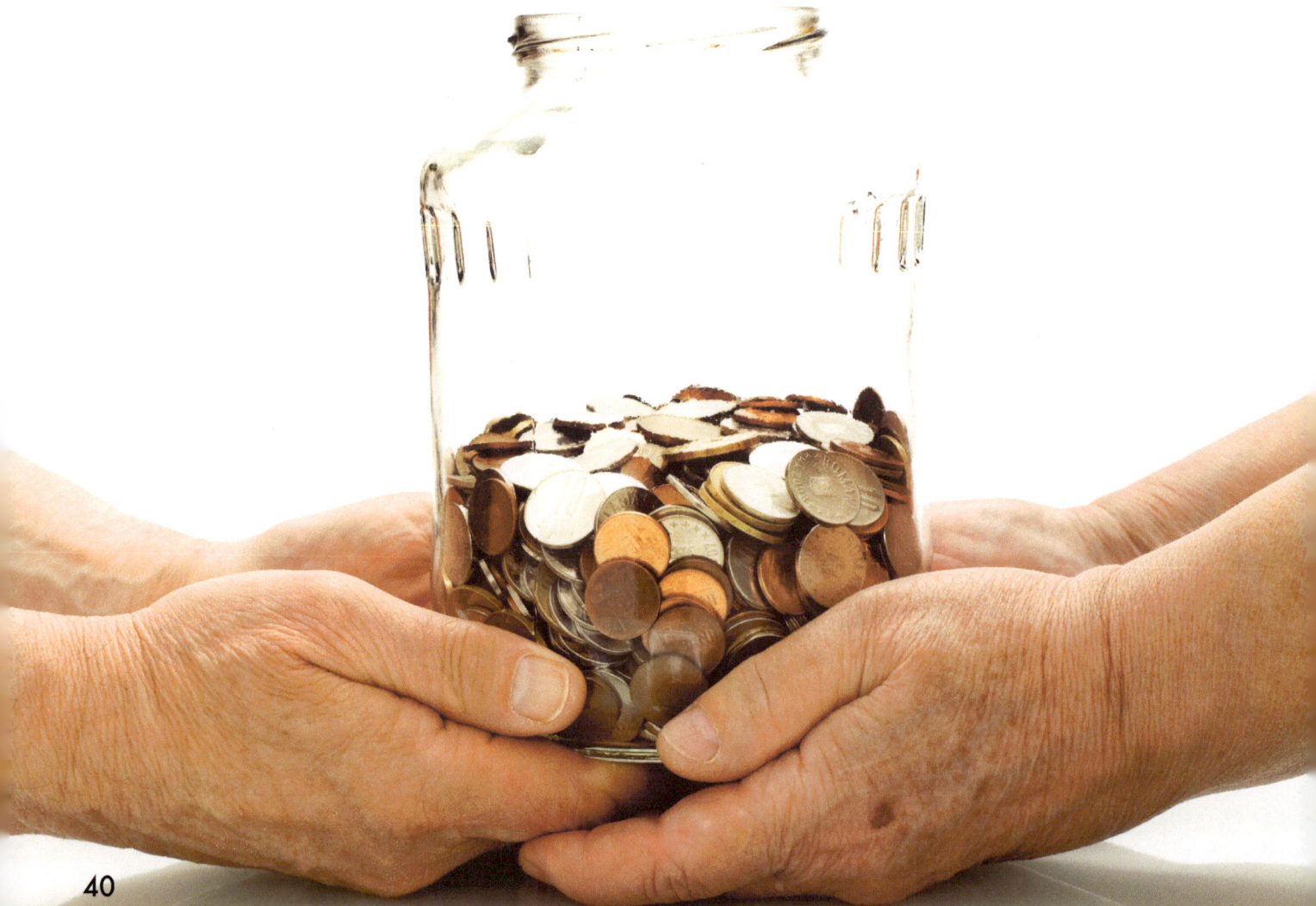

of the individual and family. Medicare and most insurance companies will pay for care following an illness, injury, or treatment which requires care delivered by licensed, trained professionals and is prescribed by a doctor. This may be considered skilled level care, that which is short in duration and aligns itself with set goals and emphasis on return to baseline with the individual or family taking over the care. Many insurers have a cap or end date of when services will become the responsibility of the individual and have a graduated process for assigning co-pays prior to the date coverage expires or ends.

Even if care services are paid for initially through insurance, it is prudent for the individual to plan for the day when they will be financially responsible for their own care needs.

Long term care is expensive.

Consider the cost of care in a long-term care setting. An assisted living averages $46,000-$70,000/year with nursing home facilities averaging $245 per day. With the cost of care sometimes exceeding $100,000 per year, those needing frequent, daily care in a long-term care facility often become financially destitute if they do not have adequate resources. Costs will vary depending on your geographic location.

Home health care is often the most preferred long-term care setting. Most Americans prefer to Age In Place in their own home. Individuals and families are often shocked to learn this can be the most expensive option. Depending on the geographic location, hourly rates for home health aides can average $23.00 to $26.00 per hour.

Let's review a typical scenario. An adult child provides unpaid caregiving to their older adult parent in their own home. The adult child has a job or career so they need someone to cover for them at the home for 10 hours per day. This timeframe allows for them to get ready for work, travel for work, work 8 hours, and travel back home. Hired help is brought in from an agency with the hourly rate at $23/hour, for 10 hours, 5 days per week. At $230.00 per day, the current expense of the family for long term care services is approximately $4,600 per month. The adult child has ensured funding is set aside, or allocated, for these care needs. The money set aside is at least $56,000 per year but set up to allow for emergencies and support as needed. There is also extra money set aside to account for mileage expense, off shift or holiday charges by the home health agency. Ideally, the allocation for yearly expenses related to long term care is $56,000-$75,00 at the current level. If the adult child was not able to provide the same level of support for some reason, such as an unexpected illness or career change, the older adult parent may have to hire 24-hour care. This too, will depend on the on-demand needs of the individual. On demand needs are those which may occur at any time throughout a 24-hour period, with no set timeframe or expectation. It is important to truly understand what the needs are and plan accordingly. Care which is required 24 hours per day due to on demand needs can be difficult to achieve in the home setting if not strategized effectively. 24-hour care in the home often exceeds $110,000 per year if provided 7 days per week. This situation will often create a need to plan for a transition to a more cost-efficient setting, such as assisted living facility. These settings offer 24-hour care at a rate which is more affordable for most individuals, further driving the demand for assisted living facilities and other long-term care settings in communities across the nation.

Now that you have a better understanding of the cost of long term care let's focus on the potential payor sources for long term care. There are some options for obtaining coverage or financial assistance for personal care assistance home health. It is important to note this information and the advice provided does not exclude the need to consult with a financial planner, advisor, or attorney. Situations can be complex with many variables, especially related to finances. Policies, regulations, industry and laws change frequently which makes it difficult to provide a true representation for every person.

Potential options for financial assistance with long term care & general summary of each:

- **Long term care insurance**
  - o Must be an eligible beneficiary or member (already have long term care insurance)
  - o Claims are processed with an emphasis on determining eligibility through a comprehensive, often tedious, evaluation period
  - o Benefits will depend on each individual policy
  - o Caps or end dates of coverage are typical
  - o Per diem coverage often does not cover 100% of costs
  - o Deductible, out of pocket expense typical during first 60-90 days
  - o Declining industry due to high cost of care and associate risks
  - o May improve financial sustainability
  - o Allows individuals to remain in their own home longer
  - o Requires physician statement

- **Veterans Administration benefit pension for eligible Veterans**
  - o Pension benefit for eligible Veterans
  - o Financial need based
  - o Complex process requiring many documents
  - o Coverage typically covers in-home or assisted living services
  - o Limited in availability
  - o Helps Veterans remain in their own home
  - o Covers spouses in some cases
  - o Individuals often need to supplement the coverage with out of pocket expenses

- **Medicaid**
  - o Financial need based
  - o Complex process for most
  - o Takes a long time to process, sometimes up to 2 years
  - o Potentially long waiting lists
  - o Coverage may be limited for in-home support

- **Charitable organizations**
  - o Grants or other financial assistance
  - o Limited availability
  - o Limited funding
  - o Application process moderately complex: Simpler but with multiple steps
  - o Supplements personal finances
  - o May be limited to specific disease type or only available for individuals with certain conditions
  - o May or may not require physician statement or confirmation of need and diagnosis.

If you think you or your loved one may qualify for one of the above entitlements or benefits, it is important to learn as much as you can and initiate the process when appropriate. Consultation with a long-term care planning specialist may assist you in knowing the right time to apply for help or assist with the application process.

Your financial portfolio and the great debate: Spend down of assets

Most of us have heard stories of individuals trying to qualify for Medicaid by spending down the assets they have accumulated. The basic principle is for individuals to spend their own money to qualify for assistance once their assets are drained. Individuals and their families should anticipate paying for their own care if they need it and especially if they have the funds to do so. In fact, if an insurance, such as Medicaid, were to pay for your long-term care for you while you still own your house it is likely you would need to pay them back once your house sold.

Nothing should be expected for free or without a condition when it comes to the expense of long term care.

Medicaid was designed to assist older adults with their care as they age and require a nursing home. Humans have never lived longer, often with more complex disease states or co-occurring chronic conditions than ever before. The demand for financial assistance through the Medicaid long term care program is very high with some states experiencing long delays in processing applications and long wait lists once someone is approved. It is the responsibility of individuals and families to be prepared financially and have a plan, regardless of your income or financial portfolio.

What is your financial portfolio?

One of the most important questions is how much cash do you have? This is forward and direct but this is what we need to look at.

- If you needed to pay for care suddenly, would you have enough cash to pay for it?
- Are assets needing sold or liquidated and how long will it take?
- How can assets be re-allocated or set-aside for future use specifically for long term care?

It's never good to have to beg a home health agency to continue services while you cannot make payment. In fact, in most states it is customary for agencies to require a down payment prior to the start of services. It is important to consider just how much cash you may need on hand and how to obtain it without delay. Ensure assets can be converted to quick cash for immediate funding, if necessary. Don't wait for a crisis to liquidate assets that must be sold to generate cash.

What about transfer of funds to reduce your personal portfolio?

Some individuals choose to transfer their assets instead of liquidating them, which may include actual hard assets such as vehicles or real estate or retirement accounts. Transfer or protection of assets is complicated and needs to be completed with consultation of the appropriate professionals. Meeting with a financial planner or advisor is recommended for those who need help reviewing their portfolio and understanding the best plan for financial readiness. Each state will have their own set of regulations and guidelines for preparing your assets and may offer tips for long term care planning.

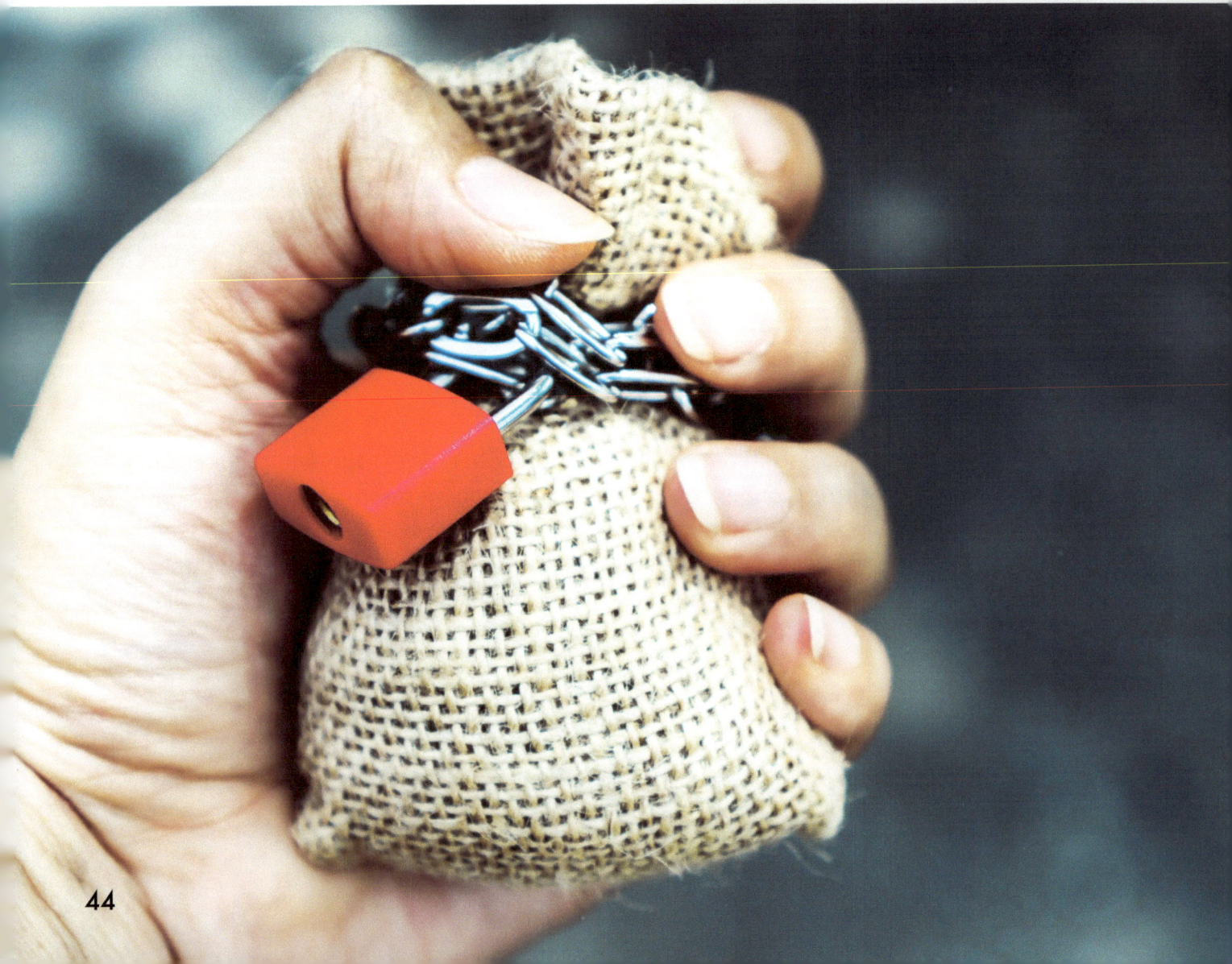

Attorneys who specialize in estate planning can assist with trusts or other documents. It is important to understand laws and customs pertaining to healthcare and financial decisions as well as how an estate is managed by someone else will depend on each state.

Your financial portfolio review should also include liabilities such as debt and monthly expenses, including medical, utilities, rent/mortgage, food, gas and more. Once it is anticipated your monthly expenses for medical will exceed your monthly income, it is vital to act quickly and determine the best course of action. Long term care facilities will not allow individuals to remain in their facility if payment is not received or some confirmation of a Medicaid application in process. Home health agencies will not typically hold services. This places the individual requiring care at risk of harm due to forced situations which could have been prevented. In these situations, care is only possible through the good will of a family or friend who is not always the best choice. Frequently the older adult may be placed in a setting which does more harm than good, creating worsening health and wellbeing while potentially increasing health care costs.

Planning for long-term care is highly personal and the responsibility of each individual.

NOTES:

Complete your financial portfolio to understand your assets and liabilities:

Assets or Resources

Types of Monthly Income:

	SELF	SPOUSE
• Pension or Retirement Benefits	_____	_____
• Dividends or Interest	_____	_____
• Supplemental Security Income (SSI)	_____	_____
• Social Security Disability	_____	_____
• Social Security Retirement or Survivor Benefits	_____	_____
• Railroad Retirement Benefits	_____	_____
• Veteran's Benefits	_____	_____
• Worker's Compensation	_____	_____
• Other non-work Income	_____	_____

Est. Totals _____

Other Assets:

	Estimated value
• Residence/Home	_____
• Real Estate/Other property	_____
• Vehicle	_____
• Vehicle	_____
• Other motor equipment which titles are held	_____
• Burial Plot	_____
• Artwork	_____
• Antiques	_____
• Other	_____

Est. Totals _____

Complete your financial portfolio to understand your assets and liabilities:

Liabilities or debt

Debt:

	SELF	SPOUSE
• Mortgage	_____	_____
• Credit Card	_____	_____
• Loans (Auto/Boat/RV/Student Education)	_____	_____
• Alimony/Child Support	_____	_____
• Other	_____	_____

Est. Totals _____

Expenses:

	SELF	SPOUSE
• Rent	_____	_____
• Utilities (water/gas/electric)	_____	_____
• Food-grocery	_____	_____
• Food-restaurant, eating out	_____	_____
• Insurance Premiums/Co Pays (health, life, home, etc)	_____	_____
• Auto- Insurance	_____	_____
• Auto-Fuel	_____	_____
• Other	_____	_____
• Other	_____	_____

Est. Totals _____

step 7 — EVALUATE PAID SERVICES

Hiring Caregivers

Hiring paid help may become necessary depending on the situation. This may be due to limitations with family and friends' availability or changes with their circumstances. Paid help may reduce caregiver burn-out, offer valuable professional insight, and improve a situation. Family caregivers are encouraged to have a back-up plan in case their ability to provide the necessary assistance falls through. This may happen unexpectedly and leave the family with an urgent need to obtain help and do it quickly. Hiring outside help is recommended when the situation is less than ideal or there is a lack of available or suitable assistance, placing the individual at risk due to unmet needs. Individuals may lack an adequate plan for care which may cause a decline in overall function, poor nutrition, accidents, or more frequent exacerbations of a health condition.

Caregivers should anticipate breaks and time away from their caregiving role. It should be said that those being cared for also need a break from the same caregiver. Breaks from caregiving are typically known as "respite." Respite is an older term still used today to describe a break from the usual or temporary suspension. Respite is known to improve the sustainability of a caregiver and improve outcomes, if planned accordingly. Respite breaks should be planned as routine and scheduled.

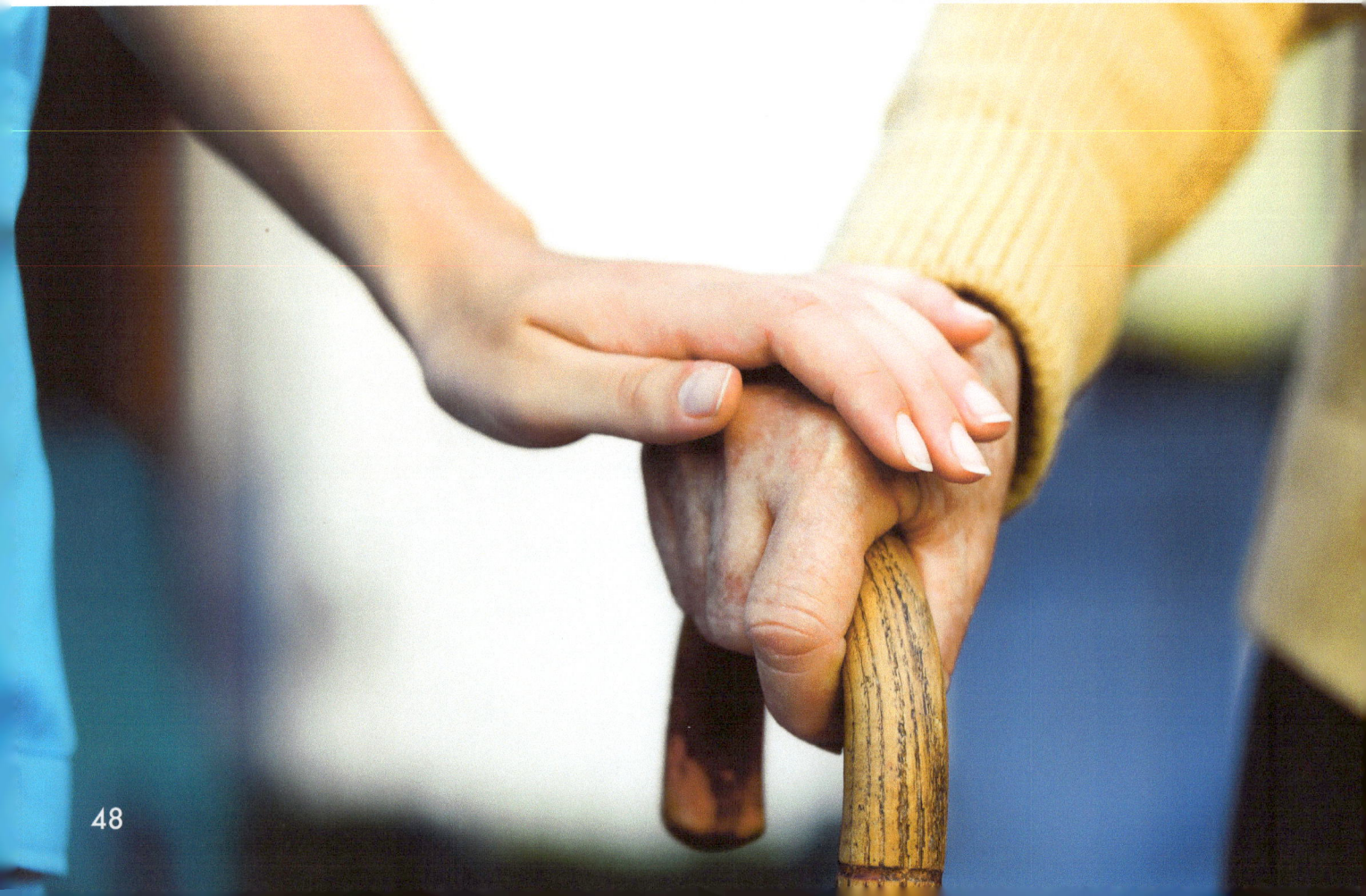

The level of assistance will vary depending on the situation. Typically, hired help meets with the individual and family to review the situation and develop the best plan for services, including scheduling.

If hiring help, it is important to have a good understanding of your needs and be very clear of your expectations. Return to Step 1 if you need to review your current needs. Understand what options are available in your community and learn as much as possible. It is important to not rush getting help on board. Choose the best option that you feel most comfortable with. It is vital for anyone with cognitive impairment to engage in developing a home health or alternative plan early. Utilize the form provided to write down available services in your community as you move through this step. Understanding what services are typically provided by paid caregivers will help in the development of your personalized home health plan.

Paid services may include:

- Assistance with Activities of Daily Living:
  - Bathing
  - Dressing
  - Toileting
  - Mobility
  - Transfers
  - Eating
- Assistance with Instrumental Activities of Daily Living:
  - Shopping
  - Housekeeping
  - Home Maintenance
  - Meal Preparation
  - Transportation
  - Setting or Making Appointments
  - Appointment Reminders
  - Social Activities & Exercise Program
  - Use of household appliances
- Medication Reminders & Compliance
- Companionship
- Safety & Security checks
- Health Maintenance
- Disease Management
- Assistance with paperwork, bills, organizing
- Supplemental staffing in a facility to help maintain current aging in place plan
- Coordination of Care
- Team based delivery of care
- Respite or breaks for caregiver/client

Services can be arranged part-time or full time and be private hire or agency. It is important to understand the differences between privately hired caregivers and agency caregivers. Privately hired caregivers are employed by the individual or family of the person needing help. Agency hired caregivers are employees of the agency and are assigned to a client using the agency protocol for intakes and new clients. Agencies charge a higher hourly rate to be able to pay taxes and provide worker's compensation insurance. They should be insured and provide appropriate training and background checks on their staff. Agencies often keep a handful of staff on hand and are often moving caregivers around depending on the needs of their clientele. Increasingly, communities are facing a geriatric workforce shortage which creates gaps and delays in services. It is necessary to allow the appropriate time for onset of services and expect to have some flexibility at times due to staffing issues. It is not unheard of to utilize two agencies at the same time to be able to fulfill a home health plan.

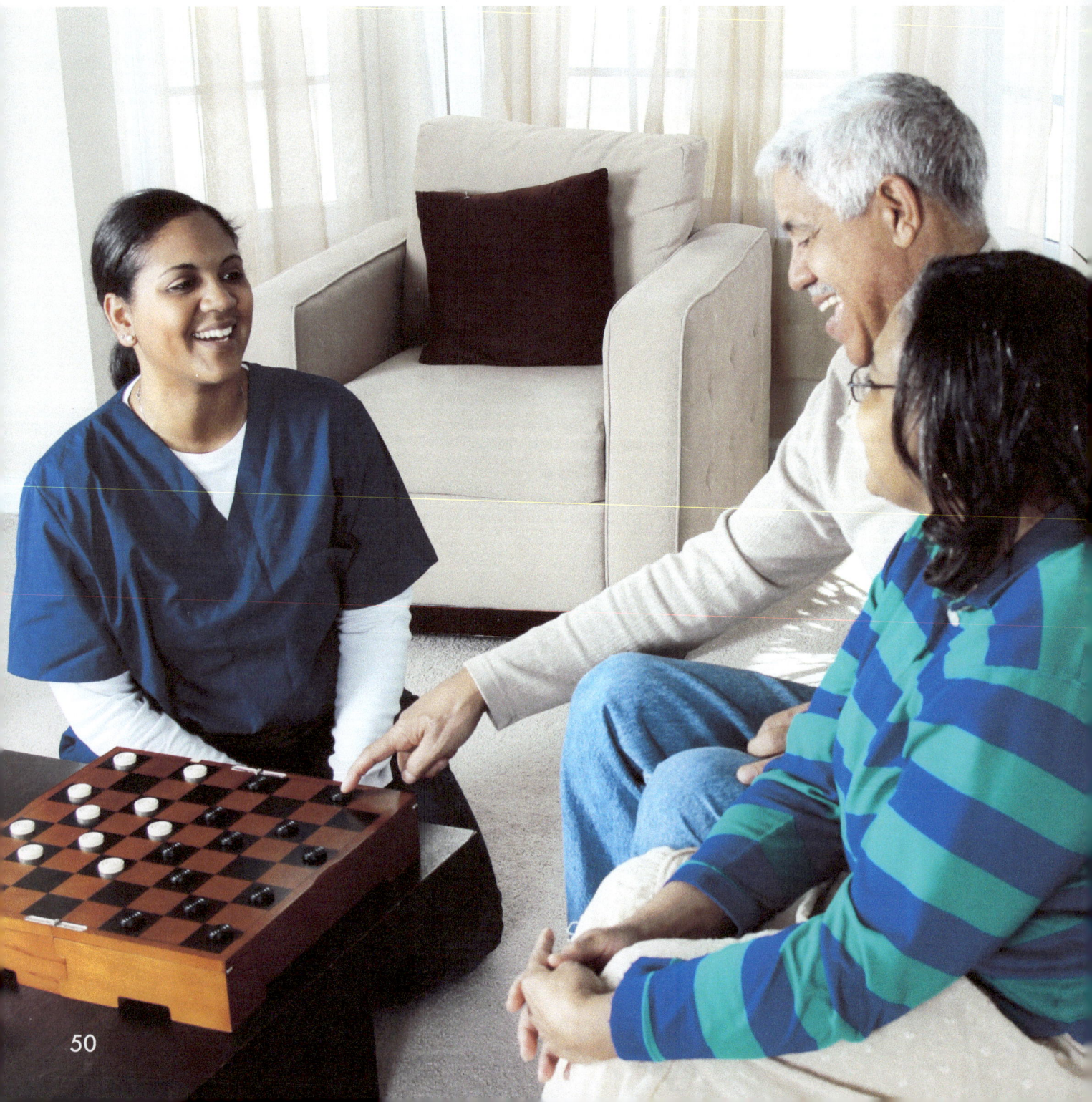

What about Private Caregivers?

Individuals who hire a private caregiver essentially become the employer of that person, necessitating a certain level of expertise and knowledge regarding payroll, taxes, and rules & regulations. Consultation with an accountant and/or attorney may be necessary.

Tips for success with private caregivers

- Know state regulations and laws
- Create a contract to be signed by all parties
- Have clear expectations
- Develop schedule to meet everyone's needs
- Have a backup plan
- Provide regular breaks
- Allow appropriate amount of down time or time off
- Have safety checks or professional oversight
- Review the home health plan regularly
- Maintain a daily log or worksheet
- Perform background check
- Check references and work history

It is important to understand the services available in your geographic location. Review your community and start to obtain a list of available services. This information is typically available through aging services, on-line resources, senior centers, phone books, health care centers or medical offices. If there is considerable distance between service providers and your location, determine if the services are available and the associated costs and fees with extra travel. Sometimes, hiring a long-term care planning specialist is helpful for finding and understanding available resources. The paid consultant can assist with ensuring a clear understanding between all parties, negotiating a contract, and provide professional oversight.

NOTES:

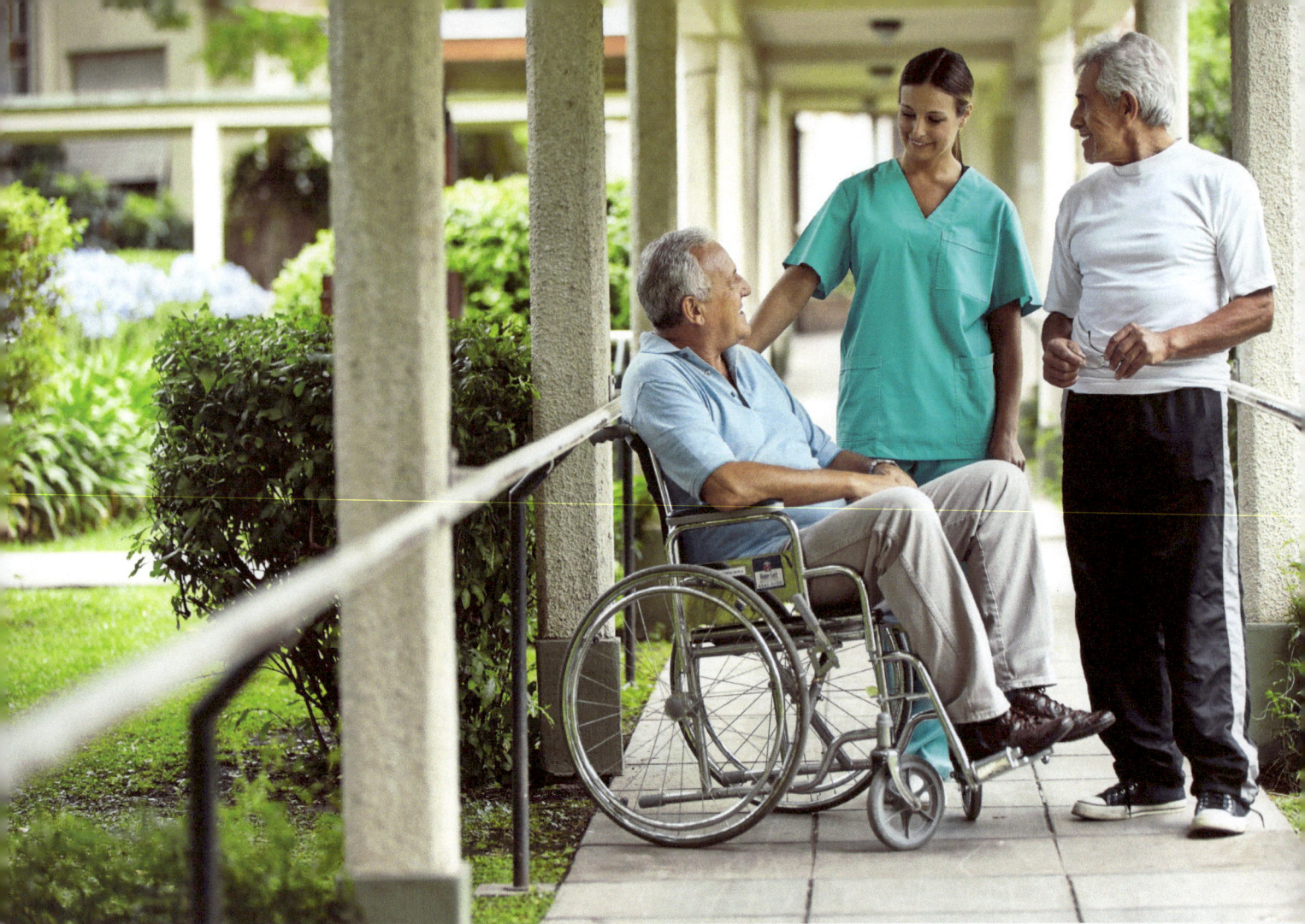

What about Long-Term Care Facilities?

Long-Term Care Facilities include:

- Nursing Homes aka Skilled Nursing Facilities
- Assisted Living
- Memory Care Assisted Living
- Adult Foster Homes
- Senior Living Communities

Some long-term care facilities are in high demand, driven by industry leaders who strive to cater to the sophisticated older adult. An individual may choose to transition to a facility if their needs can no longer be safely met at home. Sometimes the home is an additional burden with the upkeep and maintenance required. If you recall in the previous step, Step 6 - Discussing Finances, the cost of care was reviewed, emphasizing the potential impact to a person's life long savings. With the cost of care in the home setting often exceeding $200 per day for less than 12 hours of help, many choose to transition to a facility due to economics. Facilities may be as little as $150 per day and include many amenities to aid in maintaining optimal wellbeing and providing a stable environment.

The highest demand is for continuum of care communities which offer a wide array of activities and numerous levels of services. These are often referred to as senior living communities and may feature restaurants, bars, pools and spas. Nursing homes tend to be the least preferred environment but provide 24-hour care for the most complex residents who require a high level of care daily. Nursing homes, often referred to as skilled nursing facilities, are often straddled with hefty regulations and strict protocols, which may create a less than ideal environment for person-centered care. Some communities, especially frontier or rural, only have one long term care facility available. On occasion, an individual may be required to relocate out of area to find a suitable facility.

Memory support communities are popping up across America due to the steady increase in Dementia, such as Alzheimer's Disease. Newly built memory support communities are often filled before the facility reaches their 6-month anniversary. These facilities are often free-standing or attached to an assisted living. Some skilled nursing homes offer a locked unit in their facility. Individuals with Dementia may struggle to have their needs met at home due to the earlier onset of need for 24-hour supervision. It is important to have a plan in place for anyone living with Dementia. The plan should address home health assistance including a backup plan. As well as facility care, in case 24-hour assistance is no longer available. Many memory care facilities allow individuals to stay for a short duration if necessary. It is customary for the facility to review each potential client thoroughly and determine appropriateness for admission. The review process may be lengthy and based on bed availability as well as staffing.

Planning for a future transition to a facility involves researching the available services in your area and understanding the options as well as costs. Field trips or visits to the various facilities is recommended. Schedule one visit to have a tour, meet staff, and obtain valuable information. Plan a second visit as an unscheduled, unannounced visit to get an impression on your own. Keep a folder with all the handouts and brochures while utilizing the form provided to list out pros and cons and other pertinent information.

A common request includes what to look for and what questions to ask when visiting a facility. Here's some tips to help you feel prepared as you begin your research.

Things to look for in a facility:

- Cleanliness of facility
- Cleanliness of residents
- Residents engaged in activities
- Full Activity Calendar with a daily offering
- Friendliness & Attitude of the staff
- Exits & Emergency items clearly marked
- Working smoke detectors
- Nutritional & Dining area appearance
- Snack and meal choices
- Accessibility Features
- Room layout
- Odors
- Ease of access for visitors
- Administration or other office support staff availability
- Outside space

Questions you may consider asking of any facility:

1. What is your staff to resident ratio?
2. Who provides medical attention and how often?
3. How often are the care plans updated?
4. Who updates the care plans and how are residents involved?
5. What are the levels of service and what services are included with each level?
6. Do you require a bed-hold fee if bed not occupied temporarily?
7. What are your fees, including move-in costs and down payments?
8. How is access to activities provided?
9. Is transportation included?
10. What are the extra "hidden" costs?
11. What outside services can be brought in, if necessary?
12. Are staff trained and provided continuing education regularly?
13. Can personal belongings be brought in?
14. How often is the menu updated?
15. Is there a resident council and if so, how often do they meet?

NOTES:

Use this form to help you explore options available in your geographical area:

Facility Name	Location	Cost	Special Notes

Long term care planning is a dynamic process which may change with time, just as our needs sometimes change. Depending on the situation, the time necessary to complete the 7 Steps will vary. The activities and discussions involve complex decision making which may be emotional for some. Use this guide as a foundation for helping you complete your road map for aging. Return to the 7 Steps regularly to update your information or that of a loved one.

The advice provided in this book does not exclude the need to consult with a professional, such as an attorney, financial advisor, long-term care planning specialist or medical provider. The author and 7 Steps hold no responsibility or liability for the use of the information provided nor the outcome of any individual's long-term care plan. The information found in this book are the views, thoughts, and opinions which are based on professional experience of the author. Learning styles and preferences vary depending on the person.

NOTES:

NOTES: